ATLAS
ON
DERMATOLOGY

ucb Pharma

D/1994/5.541-1
ISBN: 2-87301-010-X
©UCB Pharmaceutical Sector - Braine-l'Alleud - Belgium

Responsible editor: Diane VAN MOERBEKE
                     Chemin du Foriest
                     B-1420 Braine-l'Alleud

Lay-out: Dino Drusi Communication

Printing: IMPRIMERIE CALIFICE - B 6060 GILLY

CATHOLIC UNIVERSITY-LOUVAIN

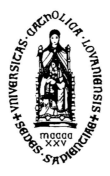

Jean-Marie **LACHAPELLE**
Professor in Dermatology,
University Hospital Saint-Luc, Louvain-en-Woluwé
and University Hospital Mont-Godinne

Dominique **TENNSTEDT**
Consultant,
University Hospital Saint-Luc,
Louvain-en-Woluwé

Liliane **MAROT**
External consultant,
University Hospital Mont-Godinne

INTRODUCTION

Dermatological theses, summaries and abstracts are legion. Some are illustrated with colour or black and white photographs, some not.
An atlas serves a quite different purpose. It is intended as an additional reference tool accessible at any time to healthcare professionals. For the consultant dermatologist it is a useful *vade mecum*. Used judiciously, it can sometimes help overcome certain patients' scepticism about a diagnosis they find difficult to accept. For the medical student it is a visual aid to help him come to grips with the more arcane aspects of this particular discipline.

In view of its size on the one hand and, on the other, the susceptibility of nosological classifications to change from time to time, this atlas is not divided into any clearly definable chapters. The choice of illustrations is also to some extent arbitrary.

We wish to express our warm thanks to UCB-Pharma: without their support, the production of this atlas would not have been possible.

J.M. Lachapelle

TABLE OF CONTENTS

BASIC LESIONS

From its beginnings dermatology has been a morphological discipline, sustained by a diagnostic process depending mainly on the interpretation of lesions appearing on the skin and mucosa.
Various attempts at classification of dermatoses were made in the 19th century. Alibert's "Two centuries of dermatology" is a fine illustration of these.
In time the diagnosis came to be based increasingly on an analysis of the "basic lesions" (e.g. bullae) or of the "associations of basic lesions" (e.g. papulopustular lesions) present or absent in the individual case.
By adopting this morphological approach dermatologists thus attempted, perhaps unconsciously, to cover up the inadequacy of their knowledge of aetiology and pathogenesis.
Times have now changed, and the causes and mechanisms of many skin diseases have been clarified in whole or in part. In line with this, modern dermatology textbooks include chapters concerned with an aetiological and/or pathogenetic classification, yet analysis of the basic lesions must remain the instinctive first step in all diagnostics: it is to the practice of dermatology what the tonic sol-fa is to music. Firmly imprinted on our minds, it must be harmoniously combined with modern investigations of internal-medical nature to reach a more exact diagnosis.
It is in recognition of this situation that a description of the principal basic lesions is presented in this atlas.

* LACHAPELLE J.M., TENNSTEDT D., DEGREEF H., DE BERSAQUES J., de la BRASSINNE M.
  Two centuries of dermatology. Jean-Louis Alibert. Ed. Glaxo, Brussels, 1994, 200 pages.

MACULES

A macule is a non-infiltrated mark which differs in colour from adjacent skin.

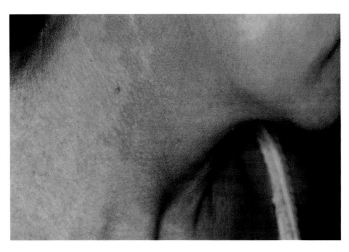

ERYTHEMATOUS MACULE

The skin coloration varies from pale pink to dark red and disappears on vitropression. It is the result of more or less intense vasodilation (e.g. blushing from modesty).

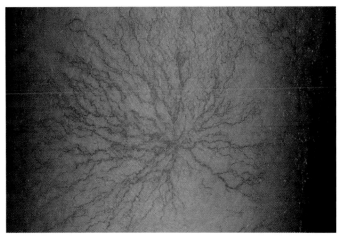

VASCULAR MACULE

These permanent marks, which disappear partially or completely on vitropression, result from the presence of an abundant network of dilated vessels in the superficial dermis (e.g. telangiectasia).

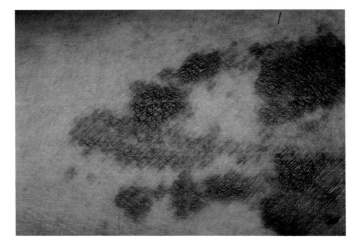

PURPURIC MACULE

The red macules do not disappear on vitropression. They are the result of extravasation of blood into the dermis (e.g. Bateman's purpura). Their colour changes in time from red to ochre.

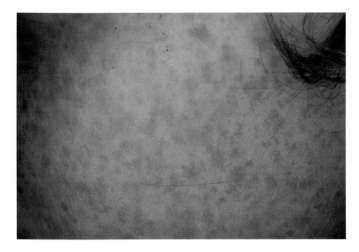

PIGMENTARY MACULES
Pigmented macules
varying in size, their colour ranging from ochre to dark brown, corresponding to melanin hyperpigmentation in the epidermis (e.g. freckles).

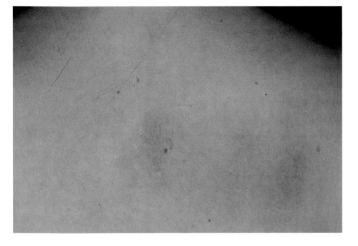

Blueish-grey macules are the result of melanin deposits extending more or less deeply into the dermis (e.g. paresthetic notalgia).

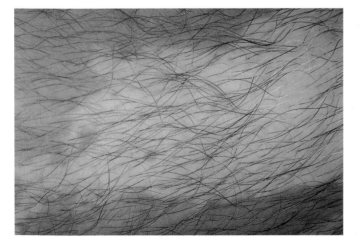

Achromic macules are white marks, varying in shape and size, which result from a decrease in the melanin content of the epidermis (e.g. vitiligo).

PAPULES

Papules are more or less well demarcated elevations of varying size. There are 3 papule types:

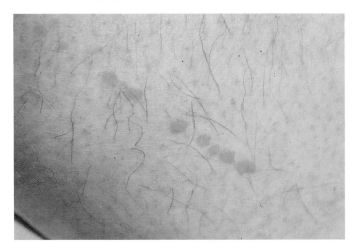

Epidermal papules
These correspond to global thickening of the epidermis (e.g. plane warts).

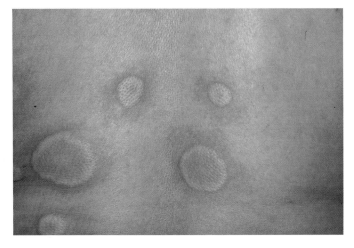

Dermal papules
These correspond to oedematous, inflammatory, or proliferative thickening of the dermis (e.g. the weal of urticaria).

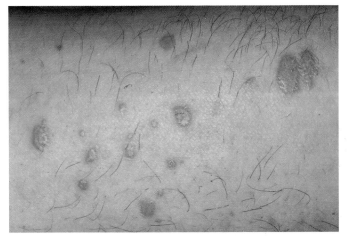

Dermo-epidermal papules
These correspond to a mixed thickening of the epidermis and dermis (e.g. lichen planus).

NODULES

Nodules are hemispherical elevations caused by inflammatory and oedematous infiltrations of the deep dermis and subcutis (e.g. rheumatoid nodule).

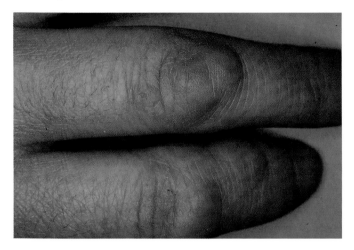

TUBERCLES

Tubercles are solid, prominent, circumscribed formations, superficially encased in the dermis. They sometimes ulcerate in the course of their development (e.g. lupus vulgaris [tuberculosis]).

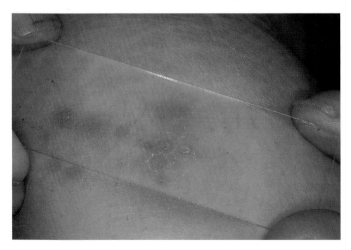

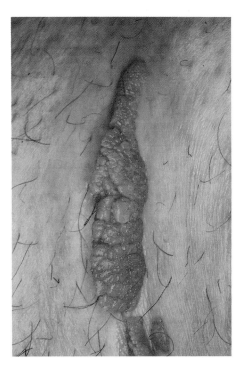

VEGETATIONS

Vegetations are filiform or lobulate excrescences, generally of soft consistency (e.g. condylomta acuminata).

WARTS

Warts are vegetations covered with a more or less thick horny layer (e.g. common wart).

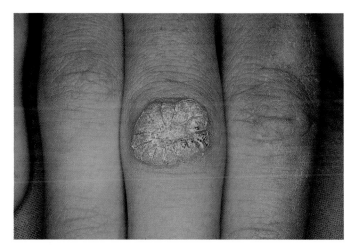

KERATOSES

Keratoses consist of epidermal lesions characterized by a localized accumulation of keratin (e.g. cutaneous horn).

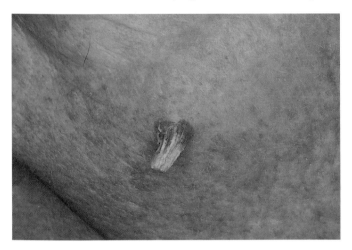

VESICLES

Vesicles are small cutaneous protuberances with a central cavity containing clear liquid. They are often hemispherical and their centre can be depressed (e.g. varicella).

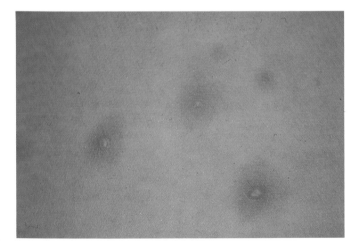

BULLAE

Bullae are more voluminous elevations with a central cavity containing a clear, cloudy, or haemorrhagic liquid. They vary in dimensions and in tension: flaccid or firm bullae (e.g. bulla of a thermal burn).

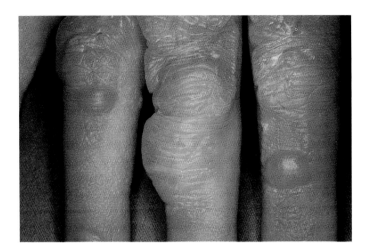

PUSTULES

Pustules are protuberances which vary in size and have a central cavity containing a purulent liquid.
They occur as primary lesions or develop from vesicles or bullae (e.g. palmoplantar pustulosis).

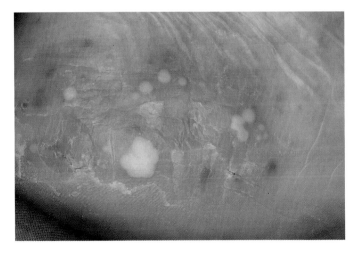

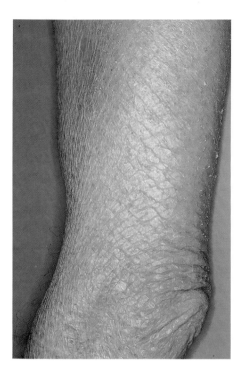

SCALES

Scales are aggregates of more or less dry horny cells formed by the superficial layers of the epidermis. They detach in fragments of varying size (e.g. ichthyosis).

CRUSTS

Crusts are concretions of fairly hard consistency which result when exudative, haemorrhagic, or purulent lesions dry out (e.g. impetigo).

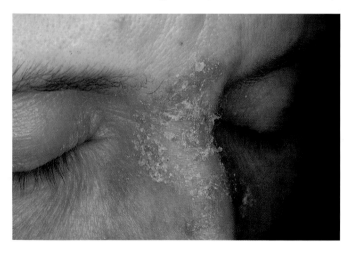

EXCORIATIONS (OR ULCERATIONS)

Excoriations are very superficial wounds. The dermis is exposed (e.g. excoriations caused by scratching).

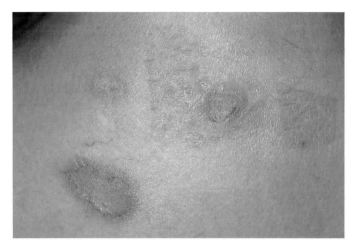

FISSURES

Fissures are linear ulcers, with or without marginal hyperkeratosis, which break through the superficial dermis (e.g. athlete's foot).

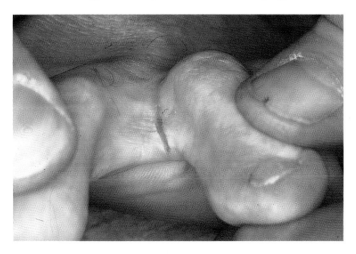

ULCERS

Ulcers are more serious losses of substance, which penetrate deep into the dermis (e.g. slough).

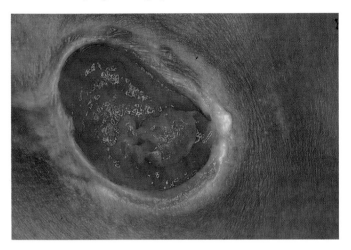

GANGRENE

Gangrene is tissue necrosis associated with loss of arterial or arteriolar blood supply (e.g. frostbite).

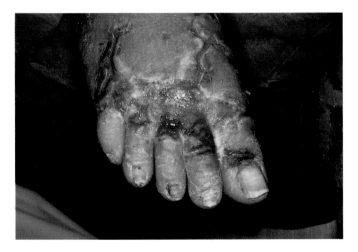

ATROPHY

Atrophy consists of a reduction in skin thickness with loss of its firmness and elasticity (e.g. senile atrophy).

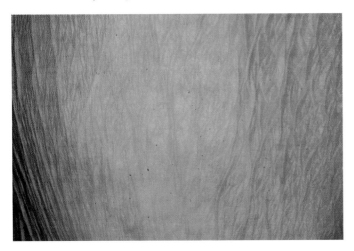

SCARS

Scars are due to modifications of the dermis or epidermis and are a sign of a variable degree of fibrosis. They are the evidence of repair of a wound or of a loss of substance (e.g. scar after a burn).

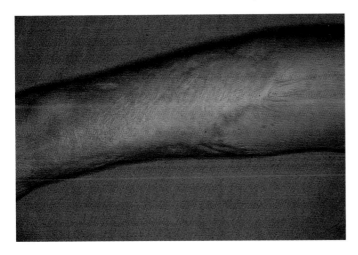

SCLEROSIS

Sclerosis means induration of the skin, which loses its normal suppleness. It is associated with coalescence of fibres in the dermis (e.g. morphoea).

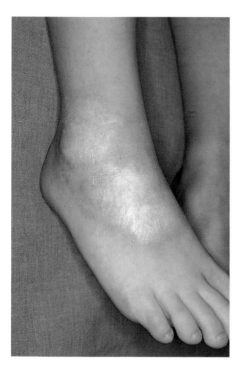

ECZEMAS

ALLERGIC CONTACT DERMATITIS AND IRRITATION DERMATITIS

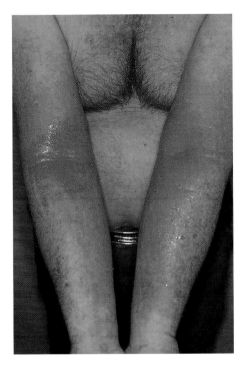

ACUTE EXUDATIVE CONTACT DERMATITIS

Acute exudative allergic contact dermatitis of the flexor surfaces of the forearms and arms after repeated application of an antiseptic lotion. Allergic reaction to hexamidine.
Countless small translucent vesicles on a background of congestive erythema, rupturing and exuding a clear serous liquid.

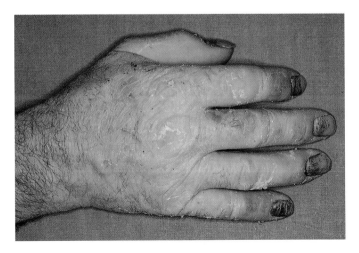

CHRONIC OCCUPATIONAL CONTACT DERMATITIS

Slightly keratotic, cracked, and infected scaly erythematous lesions of the backs of the fingers in a mason. Allergic reaction to chromium salts present in cements.

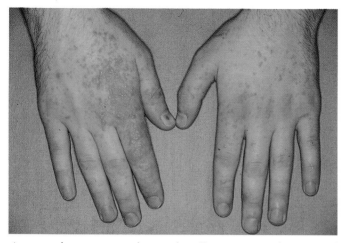
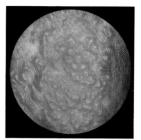

VESICULAR CONTACT DERMATITIS

Acute erythematous papulovesicular allergic contact dermatitis of the backs of the hands in a physiotherapist. Allergic reaction to the lanolin contained in a massage cream. The right hand is more severely affected than the left. The diffuse erythema, with an unsharp and fragmented margin, is covered with small translucent vesicles.

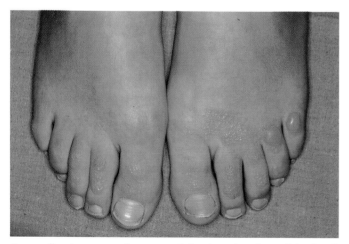
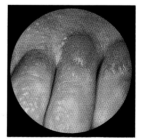

BULLOUS CONTACT DERMATITIS

Acute allergic contact dermatitis of the dorsal surface of the forefoot and toes. Allergic reaction to chromium salts used to tan shoe leather. Bullae are formed on an erythematous vesicular background.

20

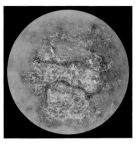

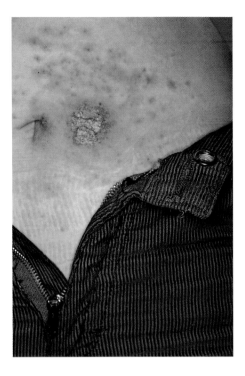

CRUSTED ECZEMA
Allergic contact dermatitis to the nickel in a jeans stud. At the point of contact there is a crusty greyish patch, partly eroded by excoriations caused by scratching. At the edges an erythematous papulovesicular eczema extends to an unclear margin.

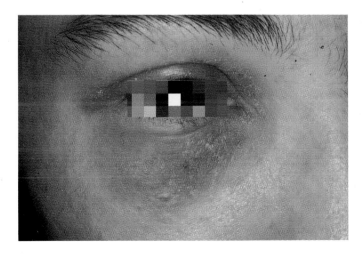

SCALY DRY ERYTHEMATOUS CONTACT DERMATITIS
Allergic contact dermatitis of the eyelids caused by the use of an antiwrinkle cream. Allergic reaction to Kathon CG®, the cream's preservative. Diffused demarcated and itchy erythematous patches of eczema with fine scales.

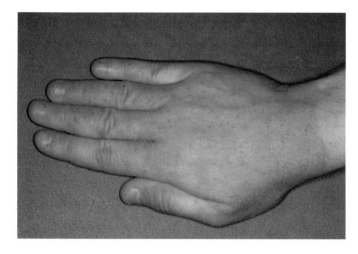

ACUTE IRRITANT DERMATITIS

Acute irritant dermatitis of the back of the hand and fingers, caused by contact with detergents. Diffuse itchy erythema. The margins of the erythema are distinct, corresponding to the zone of contact with the irritants.

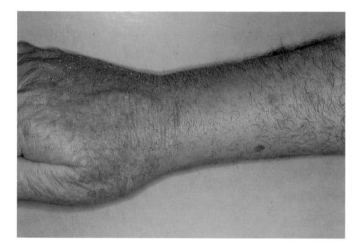

CUMULATIVE INSULT DERMATITIS OR CHRONIC IRRITANT DERMATITIS

Chronic irritant dermatitis of the back of the hand and fingers caused by contact with detergents. Scaly keratotic and chapped erythema causing pruritus and pain.

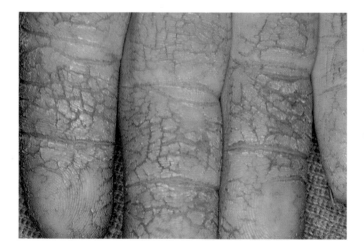

CHRONIC PALMAR IRRITANT DERMATITIS

Thick greyish or blackish keratotic patches, which are fissured and chapped. The clinical picture results from the combination of physical (friction, microtraumata) and chemical factors.

CONSTITUTIONAL ECZEMA OR ATOPIC DERMATITIS

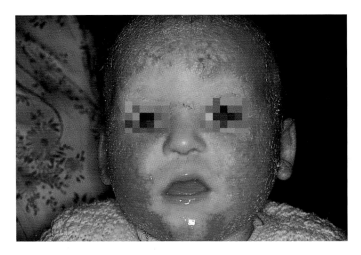

ATOPIC DERMATITIS OF THE FACE IN AN INFANT

Bright red oedematous patches of eczema with weeping vesicles.
The margins are poorly defined. The lesions predominate on the convex areas of the face: forehead, cheeks, chin.

ATOPIC DERMATITIS: INFECTED RETRO-AURICULAR DERMATITIS

Itchy exudative erythematous lesions of the retro-auricular groove, centred on a fissure at the base of the fold. Yellowish crusts are the sign of a microbial infection. These lesions, classical in childhood, can persist into adulthood.

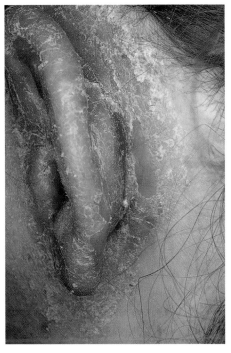

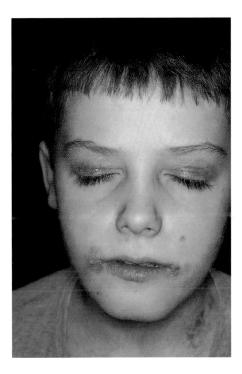

ATOPIC DERMATITIS OF CHILDHOOD

Very itchy exudative eczematous lesions of the eyelids and atopic angular cheilitis.

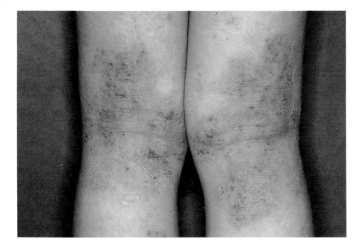

ATOPIC DERMATITIS OF THE FOLDS IN A CHILD

Lichenified and very itchy patches in the knee flexures, transversed by scratch lines. In the present case similar lesions are present in other folds (e.g. of elbows, behind the ears, under the buttocks). The lesions can persist into adulthood.

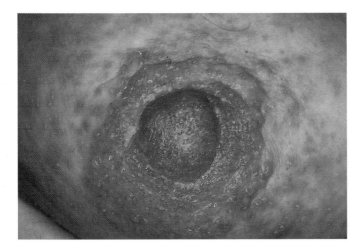

ECZEMA OF THE NIPPLES: SIGN OF ATOPIC DERMATITIS IN ADULTHOOD

Acute exudative eczematous lesions of the nipple, the areola, and the periareolar region. The lesion margins are indefinite, the pruritus intense, and the course chronic. This is a classical sign of atopy in adulthood.

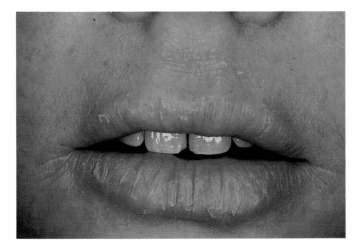

ATOPIC CHEILITIS

Atopic cheilitis affects the upper and lower lips and extends over the perioral region. Dry eczematous lesions causing chronic desquamation.

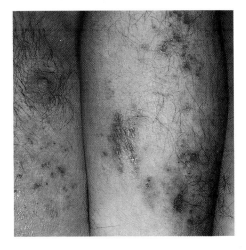

ATOPIC DERMATITIS IN THE ADULT: XEROSIS, LICHENIFICATION, AND PRURIGO

Very particular polymorphism of the lesions: skin dry and rough (xerosis), lichenified patches. There are also papules of various sizes, very strongly infiltrated, hard in consistency and often excoriated. These are prurigo papules (which used to be called "Besnier's prurigo").

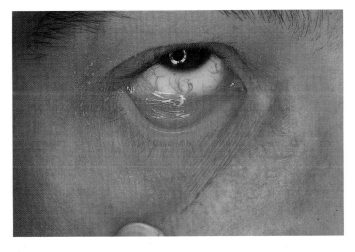

ATOPIC CONJUNCTIVITIS

Atopic conjunctivitis associated with blepharitis. This inflammation of the conjunctiva is embarrassing, sometimes painful, and often distressingly chronic. It is not unusual in the atopic adult.

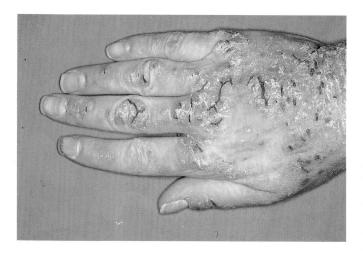

ATOPIC DERMATITIS OF THE HANDS IN THE ADULT

Chronic scaly erythematous eczema of the back of the hands. One quite characteristic feature is the irregular distribution (patchy pattern) of the lesions. Some fingers are affected, whereas others are not. The back of the hands is irregularly affected. This "disordered" topography of the lesions is frequently found in atopic dermatitis.

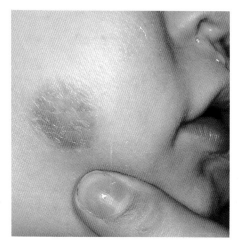

PITYRIASIS ALBA

Rounded patch of dry scaly erythematous eczema on the cheek of a child. Spontaneous healing with a tendency to transient residual depigmentation, whence the name *pityriasis alba*. It occurs more frequently in atopic patients.

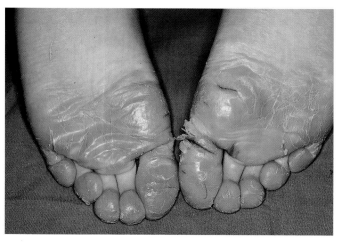

JUVENILE PLANTAR DERMATOSIS

This condition, the site of which is generally the anterior third of the sole, always bilateral, and often symmetrical, is characterized by the triad of erythema, hyperkeratosis, and fissures. The skin often has a shiny collodion-like appearance. It often becomes worse in winter and is perhaps more common in atopic patients ("atopic winter feet").

photo 1

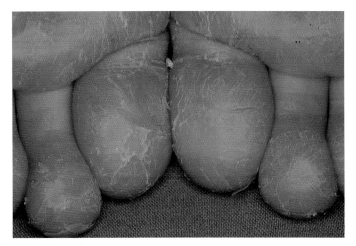

photo 2

NUMMULAR DERMATITIS (DISCOID ECZEMA)

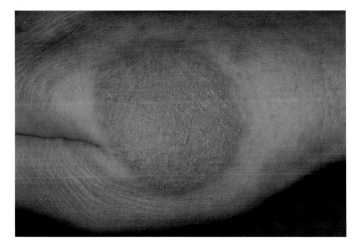

Exudative variety: round erythematous plaque (*nummulus* = coin) covered with numerous weeping vesicles which develop into small crusts.

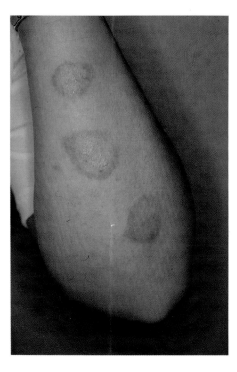

Dry variety of nummular dermatitis:
several round or oval erythematous plaques, well demarcated and isolated from each other. Their diameter varies from one to several centimetres and they are covered in fine dry scales.

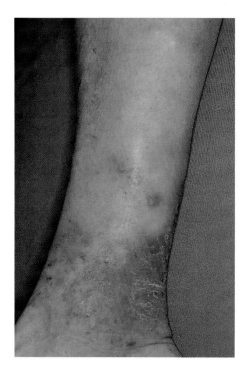

GRAVITATIONAL ECZEMA
Patches of itchy erythematous dry eczema, often accompanied by scratches. The lesions are sometimes situated along the course of varicose vessels.

SEBORRHOEIC DERMATITIS

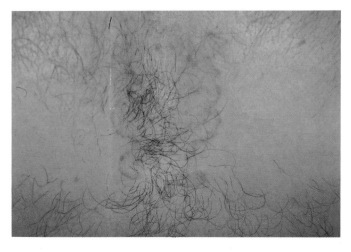

SEBORRHOEIC DERMATITIS OF THE TRUNK
Red circinate plaques in the presternal and/or interscapular region, covered in slightly itchy greasy scales. Very slight depigmentation occurs in the centre of the lesion.

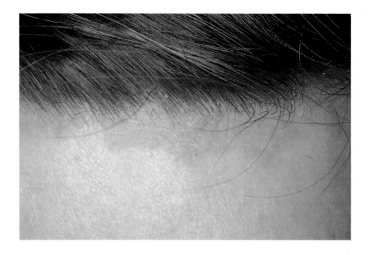

SEBORRHOEIC DERMATITIS OF THE HAIRLINE

On the scalp it is characterized by diffuse itchy erythema covered in greasy scales. The lesions sometimes spread to the forehead, as in the present case, where they form what is commonly known as the *corona seborrhoeica*: erythematous patches dotted with steatoid scales, which, following the hairline, show scalloped and arched margins.

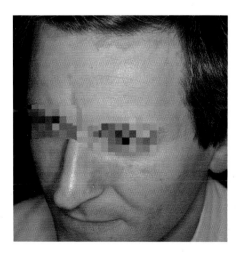

SEBORRHOEIC DERMATITIS OF THE FACE

The scaly erythematous lesions are well demarcated and have characteristic sites: hairline, nasolabial folds, vertical mediofrontal fold, and the free edges of the lower eyelids.

POMPHOLYX

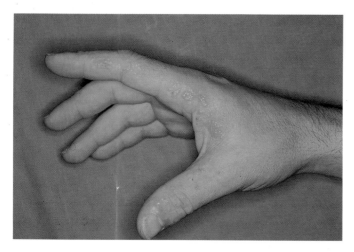

POMPHOLYX OF THE FINGERS

The vesicles of pompholyx are arranged in groups on the lateral sides of the fingers. They are hard to the touch, encased in the epidermis, translucent, and classically compared to grains of sago or to cooked tapioca. They are accompanied by intense itching.

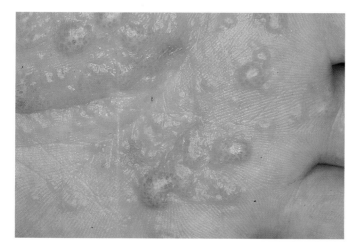

BULLOUS POMPHOLYX OF THE PALMS (CHEIRO-POMPHOLYX)

The vesicles encased in the palmar epidermis coalesce to form true bullae, which are sometimes haemorrhagic.

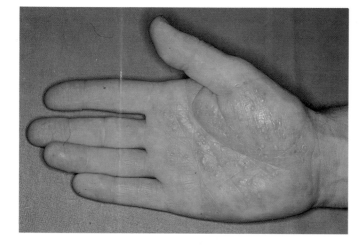

ECZEMATOUS POMPHOLYX OF THE PALMS

Eczematous pompholyx represents an association of pompholyx vesicles with scaly erythematous patches with diffuse margins.
The itching is fierce and the course is characterized by successive, even subintrant episodes.

ASTEATOTIC ECZEMA (OR WINTER ECZEMA, ECZÉMA CRAQUELÉ, OR ERYTHEMA CRAQUELÉ)

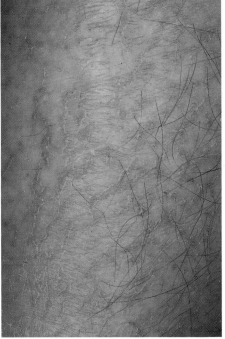

Dry eczema with imprecise margins reminiscent of crazy paving. The cracks in the "paving" correspond to fissures of variable depth, with pin-point bleeding. The name "erythema craquelé" is nowadays preferred to "eczéma craquelé".

URTICARIAS

CONTACT URTICARIAS

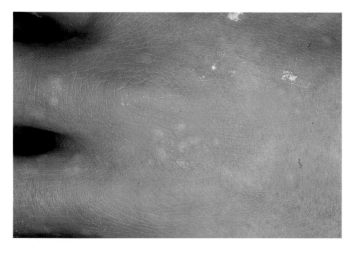

LATEX CONTACT URTICARIA

Urticarial weals occurring within minutes of putting on surgical latex gloves. These weals can spread beyond the actual site of contact because this is an immunoallergic urticaria (specific IgE are sometimes present). Generalized urticaria with systemic symptoms can therefore occur: allergic rhinitis, conjunctivitis, asthma-like attacks, anaphylactic shock, etc.

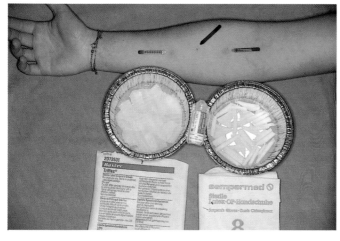

PRICK TEST WITH LATEX

Diagnosis of latex contact urticaria: the prick test is performed with a lancet, using incubation liquid from the suspected latex gloves.

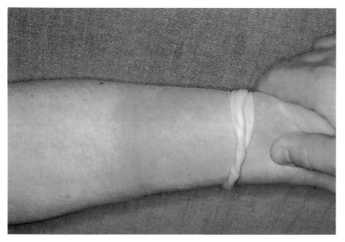

PROVOCATIVE USE TEST WITH LATEX GLOVES

In cases of doubt (prick test difficult to interpret), a provocation test can be performed, if necessary with the suspected glove. This will always be done initially with a finger-stall, which is slipped onto a moistened finger for 10 min.
The provocation test must always be done in a hospital environment.

PHYSICAL URTICARIAS

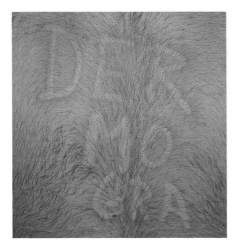

DERMOGRAPHISM
Drawing on the skin with a blunt tip produces a linear erythema with an oedematous component. The dermographism appears 5 to 10 min after the rubbing. It can be isolated or associated with chronic idiopathic urticaria.

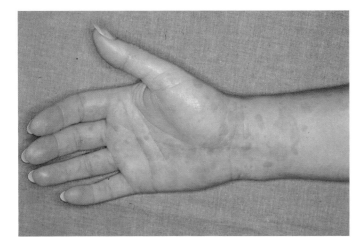

PRESSURE URTICARIA
Very itchy deep oedema occurring several hours (6 to 12 hours) after strong pressure on a precise area, e.g. on palmar side. Feet can be affected after walking, as can buttocks after prolonged sitting.

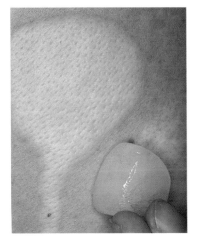

COLD URTICARIA
Eruption triggered by cold: the application of an ice-cube for 3 to 10 min systematically reproduces an urticarial weal. Nevertheless, in the present case it would be appropriate to perform a second test to eliminate aquagenic urticaria (with immersion of one hand in water at ambient temperature).

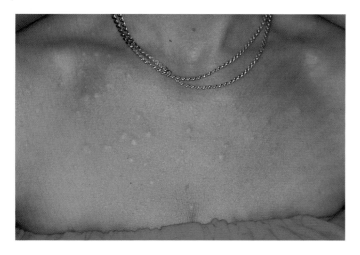

SOLAR URTICARIA

This very rare variant of urticaria occurs within minutes on exposure to sunlight. The eruption can persist for three to four hours. Photobiological investigation very easily confirms the diagnosis (photosensitivity test positive with UVA and/or UVB).

COMMON URTICARIAS (MEDICINES, FOOD, IDIOPATHIC)

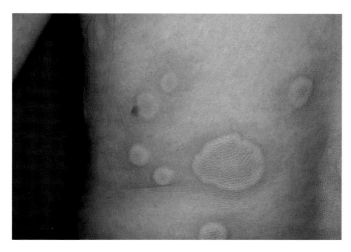

URTICATED WEALS

Eruption of oedematous urticated weals which can coalesce into broad patches. Itching is constant and can prevent sleep. This urticaria can be the first sign of anaphylactic shock.

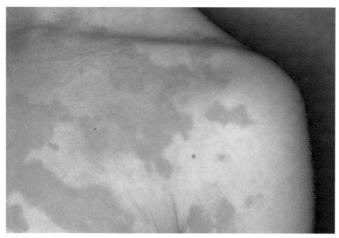

PAPULAR URTICARIA

Urticarial weals spread symmetrically over the body, most often blamed on medicines. Specific foods can sometimes trigger this type of urticaria (acute urticaria). Strawberries, shellfish, fish, certain cereals, milk, eggs, and some particular food additives are most frequently the cause. The diagnosis is based mainly on provocation tests (withdrawal and re-introduction of the suspected medicine or food).

34

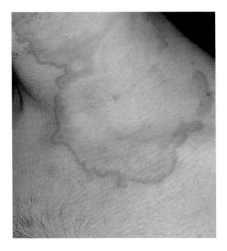

FIGURED URTICARIA

The urticarial papules describe curlicues or geographical shapes. In this case, the cause would most often be a drug (aspirin, codeine, penicillin, etc.). Again, a withdrawal test with re-introduction, if appropriate, makes it possible to reach an exact diagnosis.

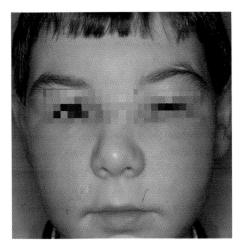

HEREDITARY ANGIO-OEDEMA

Not particularly itchy, deep urticaria mainly affecting the face (particularly eyelids and lips), the glottis, and even the larynx. This is an emergency which requires rapid therapeutic intervention (adrenaline and corticosteroids in particular). Iatrogenic causes are not uncommon.

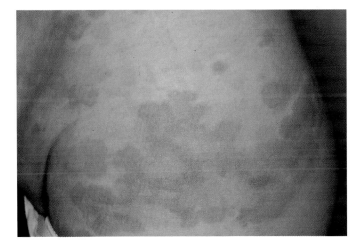

URTICARIAL VASCULITIS

Combination of urticaria with lesions of leucocytoclastic vasculitis. The urticarial lesions are more fixed than in classical urticaria. They last for 2 to 3 days and are frequently accompanied by joint pains and by fever. Reduced complement levels in blood are observed.

INFECTIOUS DISEASES
(OR REACTIONS TO AN INFECTION)

A. Viral diseases

HERPES VIRUS GROUP

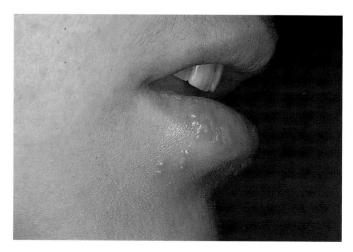

TYPE I HERPES
Herpes of the face
Multiple vesicles arranged in a cluster on an erythematous background. The lesions are usually painful and in most cases preceded by a burning or itching sensation. The vesicles rupture spontaneously after a few days and drying occurs later. Recurrences are typical (recurrent herpes), usually at the same site.

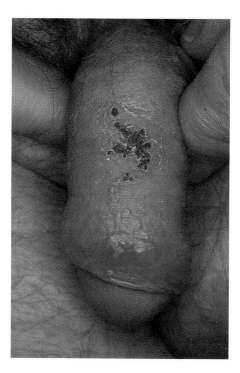

TYPE II HERPES (GENITAL)
Herpes of the penis
There are lesions which correspond to two stages of development: vesicles on an erythematous base on the prepuce (recent attack) and black crusts on the shaft (old attack). The lesions are itching and painful. The diagnosis is confirmed with liquid from a vesicle: smear for immunological diagnostics with the aid of monoclonal antibodies and culture.

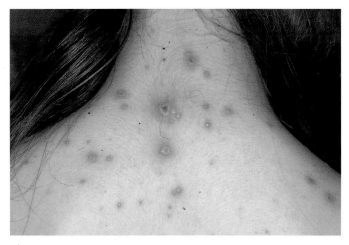

photo 1

VARICELLA - ZOSTER

Varicella and herpes zoster are associated with infection by the virus *Herpes varicellae*.

Varicella

Vesicles on a background of healthy skin or surrounded by an erythematous ring (photo 1), distinctly separated from each other, whose contents become cloudy secondarily. The central umbilication is classical. They develop to form an adhesive crust which sometimes leaves a depressed scar when it detaches (photo 2).

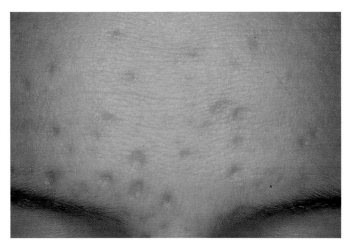

photo 2

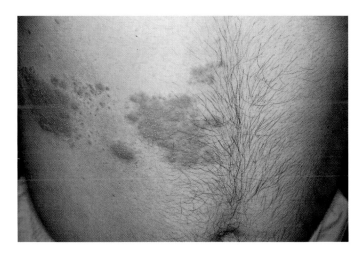

Zoster of the trunk

Vesiculobullous dermatosis preceded and very often accompanied by considerable pain (especially in old people). The lesions are strictly unilateral and correspond to the tract of a nerve root. In the present case an intercostal nerve is involved ("fiery half-girdle").

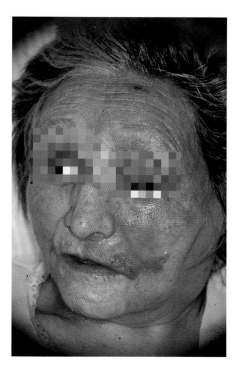

Ophthalmic nerve zoster
In the present case the topography of the lesions makes it possible to say that two branches are affected by the infectious process: the ophthalmic branch and the superior maxillary branch. The third branch, the inferior maxillary, is spared. The presence of vesicles on the nostril shows that the nasociliary nerve is involved.

PAPILLOMAVIRUS GROUP

The papillomaviruses are responsible for the occurrence of various types of benign tumour, viral warts.

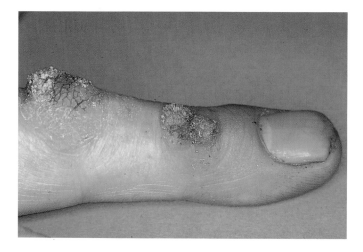

COMMON WARTS
Small greyish keratotic tumours, rough to the touch, on the backs of the fingers. Common warts are contagious and autoinoculable.

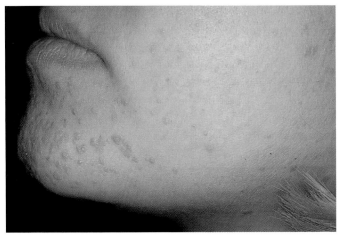
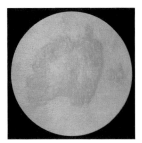

PLANE WARTS

These warts are mainly located on the face and on the back of the hands or fingers. They are orange very slightly raised papules. The linear disposition is typical (Kœbner's phenomenon caused by autoinoculation along scratch lines).

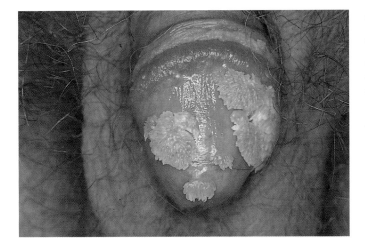

CONDYLOMATA ACUMINATA

Fleshy reddish formations on the genital organs.
Condylomata acuminata are contagious (sexually transmitted disease) and can spread rapidly.
The maceration is sometimes considerable.

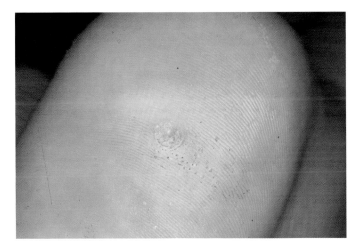

PLANTAR WART

Distinctly demarcated keratotic formation which is often deeply embedded in the skin of the sole. The disappearance of dermatoglyphics all over the surface of plantar warts is typical and makes it possible to distinguish this lesion from a corn. A single plantar wart is classically known as myrmecia.

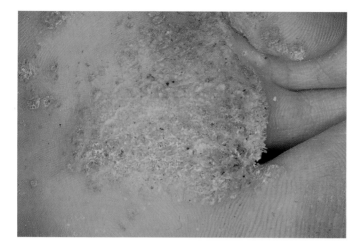

MOSAIC WARTS

Juxtaposition of numerous plantar warts forming a hyperkeratotic patch by spreading by degrees. These mosaic plantar warts are often painful (sensitivity to pressure during walking).

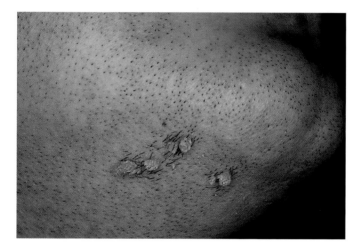

HORNY FILIFORM WART

Small pedunculate papilloma mainly affecting the face (nose, side of the neck, and cheeks). Horny filiform warts are typically found in men (shaving, especially with a razor rather than an electric shaver, contributes to dissemination).

EPSTEIN-BARR VIRUS

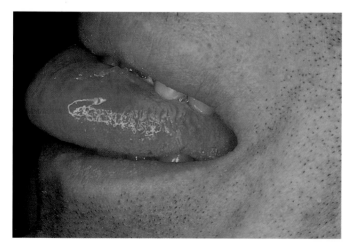

HAIRY LEUCOPLAKIA

Appearance of fine whitish striations on the sides of the tongue. Oral hairy leucoplakia is most often encountered in homosexual men suffering from AIDS. The term "hairy" is purely descriptive. The hairy appearance is associated with linear hyperplasia.

POX AND PARAPOX VIRUS GROUPS

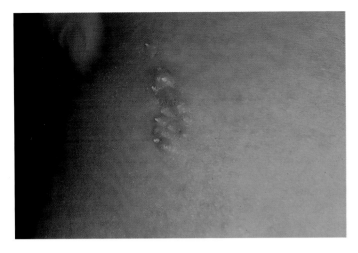

MOLLUSCUM CONTAGIOSUM

Small round papule with a smooth surface, often shiny, a few millimetres in diameter. There is often a small central depression (crater, often filled with creamy whitish material). These lesions most frequently affect children and can be secondarily accompanied by eczema around the lesion. Molluscum contagiosum is caused by a poxvirus.

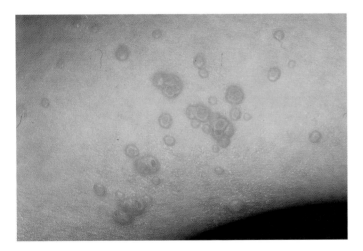

MULTIPLE MOLLUSCA CONTAGIOSA

Illustration of the phase of dissemination of the lesions. The topographical predilection for the axilla is characteristic. In some cases the mollusca contagiosa can become inflamed and there can be a superimposed infection. In adults, molluscum contagiosum is often found in the genital area. An immunological status check is indispensable in the case of very numerous lesions (especially if found on the face).

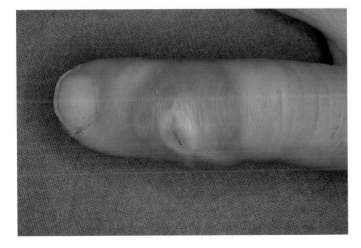

ORF

Red to violet pseudovesicular papule appearing on the dorsal face of a finger. The incubation period varies from three days to two weeks after contact with a sick animal (usually sheep). Regression without complications in about two weeks. A superimposed bacterial infection is not uncommon. Orf is caused by a parapoxvirus.

OTHER VIRUSES

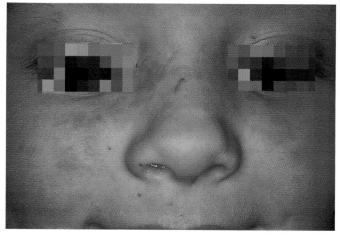

photo 1

ERYTHEMA INFECTIOSUM

Maculopapular "butterfly-wing" eruption of the face giving a puffy appearance, like "butterfly wings" (photo 1). The biphasic development of the lesions on the face is typical. After the second bout there are often numerous pink polycyclic or circinate maculopapules, describing curlicues on the limbs (photo 2). The eruption disappears in about ten days and is caused by Parvovirus B19.

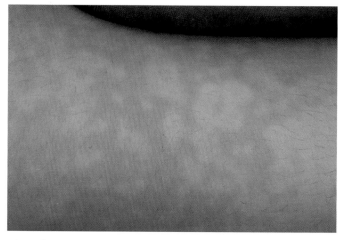

photo 2

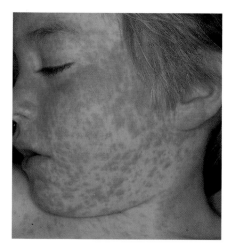

MEASLES

Maculopapular eruption, very pronounced on the face. Enanthema is also present. Some healthy skin areas can always be seen. There is often a superimposed ENT bacterial infection and injection of the conjunctivae. Measles is caused by a paramyxovirus.

HAND-FOOT-AND-MOUTH-DISEASE

Intraoral enanthema of the anterior part of the mouth, with small greyish vesicles which rupture very rapidly. The pain caused can make it difficult to eat (photo 1). Appearance of small oval vesicles about 3 to 4 millimetres in diameter on the hands and feet (photos 2 and 3). The vesicles are greyish-white and surrounded by an erythematous halo.

There is a vaguely painful sensation. Disappearance is rapid; disseminated lymphadenopathy can be present. Similar lesions are sometimes found on the buttocks. The condition is generally caused by the Coxsackie A16 virus. Other coxsackie viruses may also be responsible.

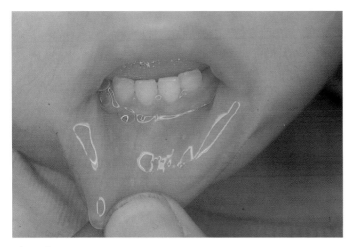

photo 1

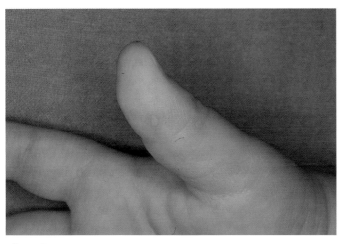

photo 2

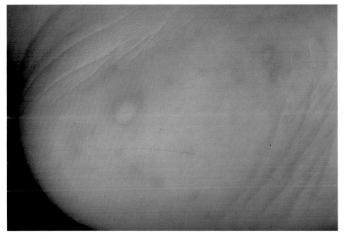

photo 3

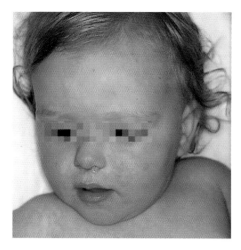

RUBELLA

Relatively modest erythematous macular eruption accompanied by suboccipital lymphadenopathy with considerable swelling.

The pale pink colour and the unobtrusive effect on general health are other features to be borne in mind. In adults and adolescents the symptoms are often more prominent (fever and more pronounced rash).

The pathogen is a togavirus.

SIGNS OF AIDS ON SKIN AND MUCOSA

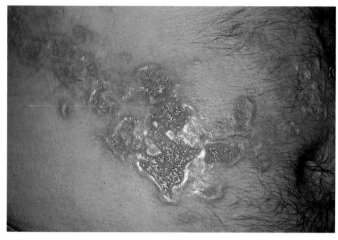

NECROTIC HERPES ZOSTER

Multiple ulcers developing from necrotic patches. These ulcerated lesions have spread considerably (photo 1) and after several weeks have left slightly atrophic cicatrized patches (photo 2).

photo 1

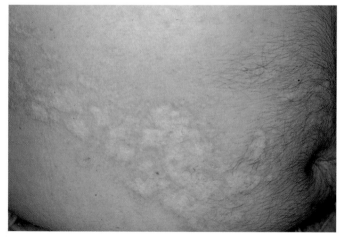

photo 2

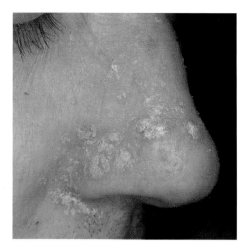

SEBORRHOEIC DERMATITIS
Seborrhoeic dermatitis, often severe and resistant to conventional treatments, can be seen in the course of an HIV infection. In the present case the involvement of the whole nasal pyramid was the first sign of HIV infection.

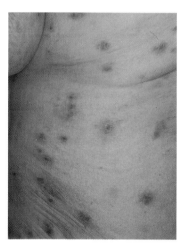

PRURIGO
In quite a number of cases prurigo-like lesions (excoriated nodules) accompanied (or caused) by diffuse pruritus are observed. The involvement of the trunk is relatively typical.

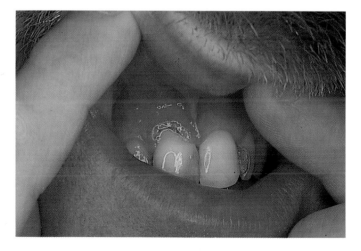

GINGIVITIS
The dentogingival junction is the site of a purulent erythema (presence of fusiform and spiral bacteria). This periodontitis is painful and shows no tendency to regress spontaneously.

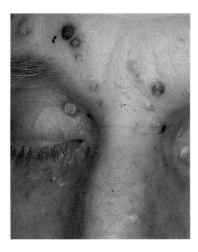

MOLLUSCUM CONTAGIOSUM

Very numerous mollusca on the face, sometimes with a few lesions which are haemorrhagic in appearance, can be seen in AIDS. The mollusca are generally very deeply embedded in the skin. Curettage is relatively difficult. The mollusca show a marked tendency to multiply.

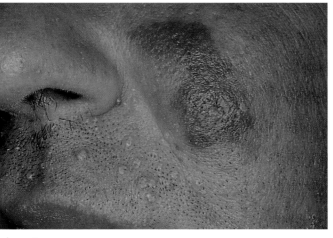

photo 1

KAPOSI'S SARCOMA

Purplish angiomatous papular lesion.
The preferred involvement of the face is typical in AIDS patients. In the present case Kaposi's nodules are observed side by side with mollusca contagiosa (photo 1). Kaposi's nodules can occur in large numbers all over the skin.
These nodules keep distinct margins with angular edges. Here again the violet colour is characteristic (photo 2). The nodules are generally completely painless.

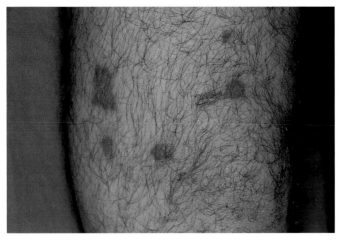

photo 2

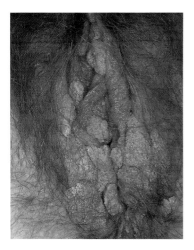

CONDYLOMATA ACUMINATA

Abnormally large or rapid spread of condylomata acuminata must always lead to a suspicion that the patient is seropositive for HIV. In the present case the condylomata acuminata spread all over the vulva and into the vaginal canal.

B. Bacterial infections

IMPETIGO

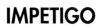

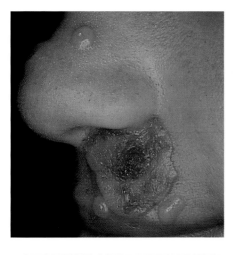

Bullous impetigo

Bullae with cloudy contents, often surrounded by an erythematous halo. These bullae rupture easily and are rapidly replaced by extensive crusty patches. Bullous impetigo is classically caused by *Staphylococcus aureus*.

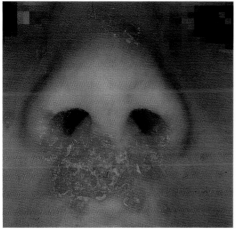

Non-bullous impetigo

Erythematous patches covered by a yellowish crust. Lesions are most frequently around the mouth. Lesions around the nose are very characteristic and require prolonged treatment. *β*-Haemolytic streptococcus is most frequently found in this type of impetigo.

ECTHYMA

Slow and gradually deepening ulceration surmounted by a thick crust. The usual site of ecthyma are the legs. After healing there is a permanent scar. The pathogen is often a streptococcus. Ecthyma is very common in tropical countries.

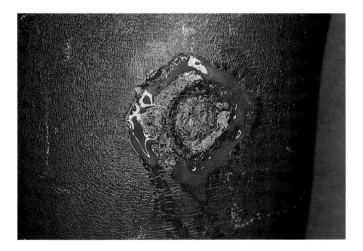

FOLLICULITIS

Inflammatory papule with a follicular pustule at its centre. The pathogen is usually a staphylococcus. Folliculitis is frequently multiple and classically located on the buttocks, thighs, or the face.

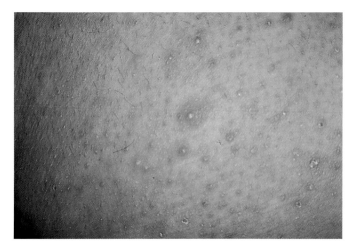

FURUNCLE (BOIL)

Acute deep folliculitis starting with a painful erythematous papule with the appearance of a central pustule. After spontaneous or induced evacuation of the pus, the furuncle often leaves a permanent scar. The pathogen is *Staphylococcus aureus*.

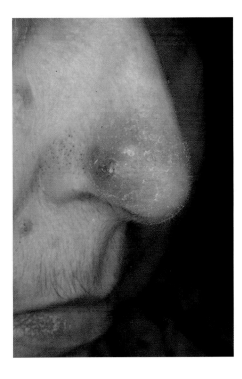

CARBUNCLE

By definition, carbuncles result from the coalescence of several juxtaposed furuncles. A large painful lump is strewn with small pustules which emerge on the skin surface.

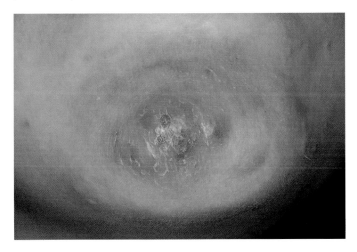

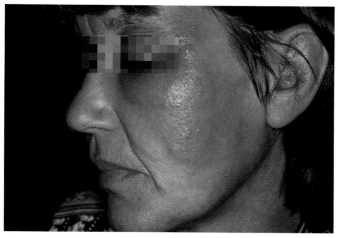

photo 1

ERYSIPELAS

Hot, painful, oedematous erythematous patches, accompanied by fever and malaise, typically caused by a streptococcus. Erysipelas can affect the face, and in this case the border against healthy skin is very distinct and raised: the "step" sign (photo 1).

On the leg one observes extensive wide patches identical with those on the face but having a less accentuated margin (photo 2). Again, the general health is affected, and there is always fever.

A mixed infection is found in most cases (gram positive and/or gram negative bacteria). There is often a portal of entry, e.g. a lesion between the toes or a wound caused by trauma.

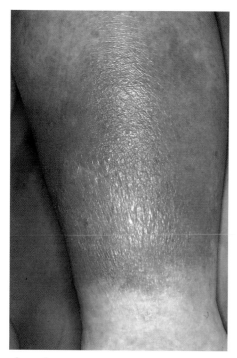

photo 2

50

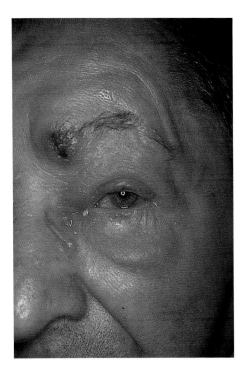

ORBITAL CELLULITIS

Deep retro-orbital infection manifests itself on the skin with periorbital oedema accompanied by malaise and fever. This is evidently a serious condition, given the possibility of spreading towards the cavernous sinus.

SEPTIC EMBOLI

Small erythematous pustular lesions occurring simultaneously in a number of places. The general context depends on the starting point of these septic emboli (cardiac involvement in rheumatic fever, gonorrhoea in the process of dissemination, etc.).

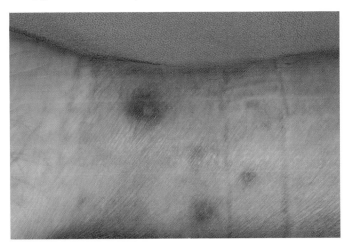

BORRELIA INFECTIONS

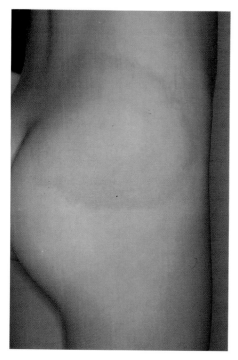

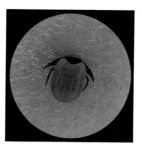

ERYTHEMA CHRONICUM MIGRANS = LYME DISEASE
Broad erythematous patch spreading outwards, with a false appearance of healing at the centre. Sometimes a small scar is found in the middle (trace of a tick bite). Erythema chronicum migrans is caused by Borrelia infection.

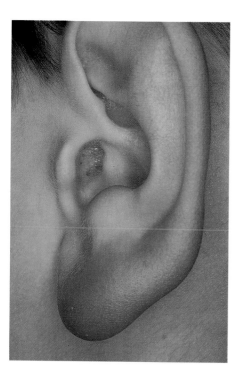

BORRELIA PSEUDOLYMPHOMA
In some cases the Borrelia infection is clinically recognized by the presence of one or more pasty nodules, mainly on uncovered parts of the body, most typically on earlobes. This type of "pseudolymphoma" is also one of the Borrelia diseases. One can include this lesion among the forms of the old "lymphocytoma benigna cutis".

PROTEUS INFECTION

In rare cases, if untreated contused lesions are present, a gram-negative microorganism such as *Proteus* or *Pseudomonas* can cause necrosis of the distal extremity of a finger.

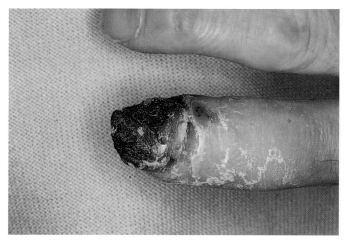

CAT-SCRATCH DISEASE

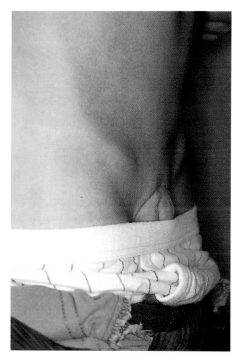

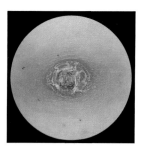

More or less fluctuant nodules with ulceration and central crust, accompanied by lymphadenopathy with considerable swelling. The young patient was scratched by his cat a few weeks previously.

INTERTRIGO

Glazed erythematous patches with the appearance of "pages of a book", centred on the base of a large fold. Maceration and infection with common microorganisms are typical.

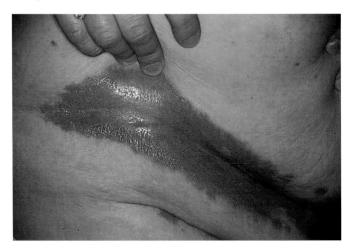

CUTANEOUS TUBERCULOSIS

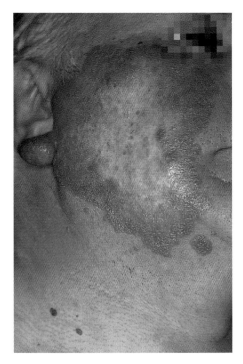

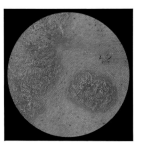

LUPUS VULGARIS

Large reddish-yellow lesion affecting the face and the earlobe. False appearance of healing at the centre. Vitropression reveals characteristic orange-red coloration, which dermatologists at the beginning of the century compared to "barley sugar", a delicacy which has now gone out of fashion.

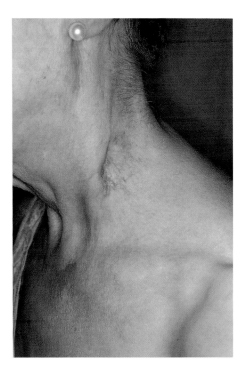

SCOFULODERMA
Chronic tuberculous cervical lymphadenopathy with skin ulceration.

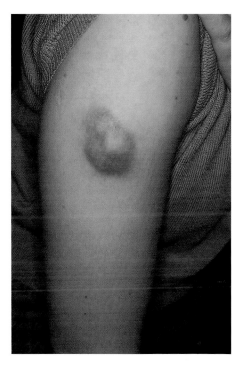

COMPLICATION OF BCG VACCINATION
Non-specific abscess formation after BCG vaccination. This complication of BCG vaccination is generally the result of an injection made too deeply.

ATYPICAL MYCOBACTERIAL INFECTIONS

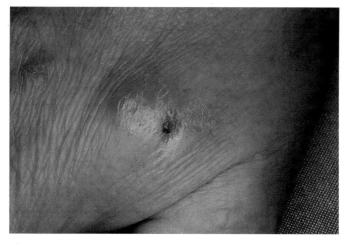

photo 1

INFECTION WITH *MYCOBACTERIUM MARINUM*

This condition is found mainly in fish fanciers (fish-tank disease) and classically appears in the form of a chain of nodules spaced like rosary beads, extending along the line of lymphatic drainage. These are more or less keratotic papulonodular lesions and/or ulcers. There is generally little pain. Deep biopsy with culture in a suitable medium very easily reveals the mycobacterium. The papulonodules can be single (photo 1) or multiple (photo 2). The latter form of the mycobacterial infection is sometimes known as sporotrichoid.

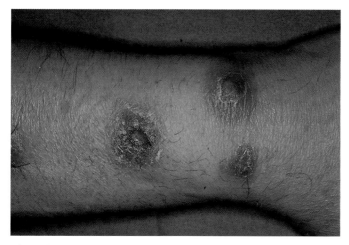

photo 2

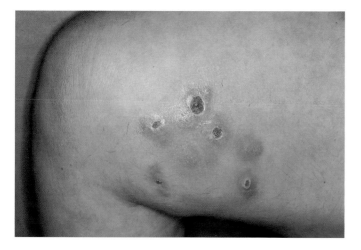

INFECTION WITH *MYCOBACTERIUM FORTUITUM* OR *CHELONAE*

Abscess and violet nodules occurring a few weeks after repeated injections as part of mesotherapy (in the treatment of "cellulitis").

CORYNEBACTERIUM INFECTIONS

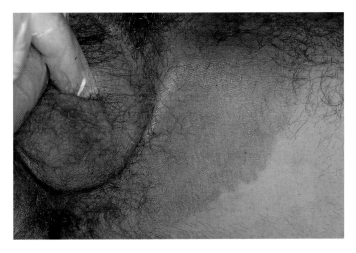

ERYTHRASMA

Broad and distinctly demarcated brownish or buff macule, with rounded margins, usually symmetrical and affecting either the groins or the axillae. These lesions are homogeneous and finely squamous. The pathogen is *Corynebacterium minutissimum*. Examination in Wood's light reveals coral-red fluorescence.

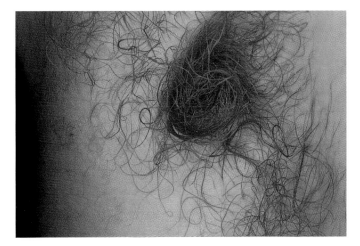

TRICHOMYCOSIS AXILLARIS

This is a bacterial infection caused by corynebacteria. The axillary hairs are surrounded by small yellowish nodules corresponding to colonies of bacteria. There is little in the way of subjective symptoms. The sweat sometimes becomes yellowish.

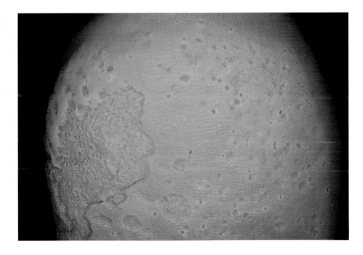

PITTED KERATOLYSIS

Small serpiginous erosions of the horny layer with a punched-out appearance, mainly found on weight-bearing areas of the soles and causing an interruption in footprints. An associated plantar hyperhidrosis is often present. The erosions correspond to areas of desquamation in a block of the horny layer invaded by corynebacteria.

C. Treponematoses and other sexually transmitted diseases

SYPHILIS

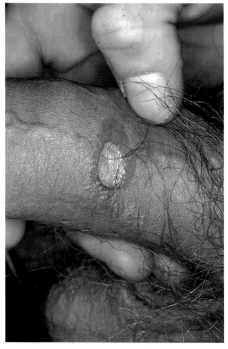

photo 1

SYPHILITIC CHANCRE (PRIMARY SORE)

Ulceration with erosion situated on the glans penis or sheath. Distinctly palpable induration. Considerable swelling of inguinal lymph nodes, usually unilateral (photo 1). In women the chancre is often accompanied by considerable oedema of the labia majora. The characteristics of female chancre (photo 2) are identical with those in the male.

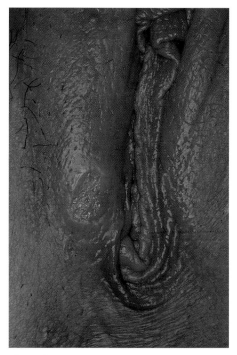

photo 2

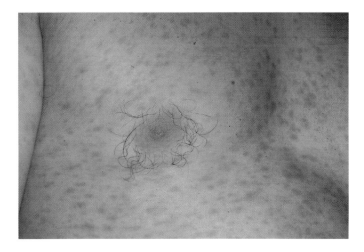

SECONDARY SYPHILIS (MACULAR SYPHILID)

Occurring about six weeks after the start of the chancre, secondary syphilis appears in the form of pink oval macules with little or no scaling and no itching. These macules are located mainly on the trunk.

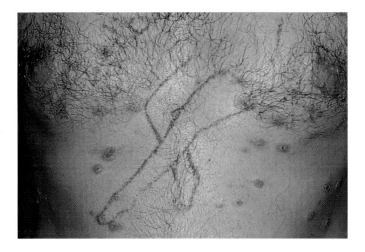

LATE SECONDARY SYPHILIS

Dull red, sometimes brownish, very distinctly indurated papules, which are not itchy, located on the trunk and on proximal regions of the limbs.

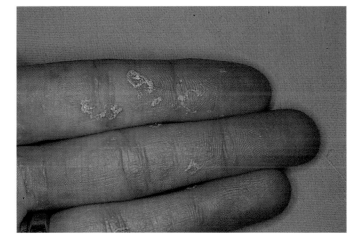

PAPULAR SYPHILIDS

Slightly reddish macules with peripheral desquamative collarette (Biett's collarette). These papular syphilids occur four to twelve months after the chancre.

GENITAL GONORRHOEA

Diffuse redness of the glans, purulent urethral discharge, considerable dysuria, pollakiuria. Presence of two mollusca contagiosa, equally sexually transmitted.

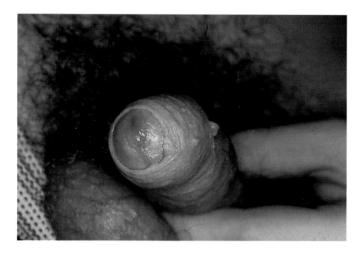

D. Mycoses

DERMATOPHYTOSES

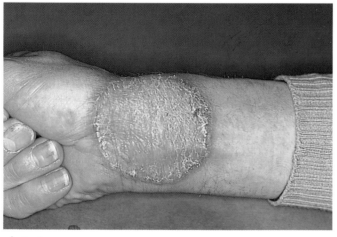

photo 1

TINEA CORPORIS

Round or oval lesion, as in the present case, with a distinctly raised margin, sometimes with fine vesicles, sometimes very scaly. There is often a false appearance of healing at the centre. These round lesions are generally slightly scaly. Pruritus is not always present as a subjective symptom. The lesions can be single (photo 1) or multiple (photo 2). The pathogen is generally *Microsporum canis* or *Trichophyton rubrum*.

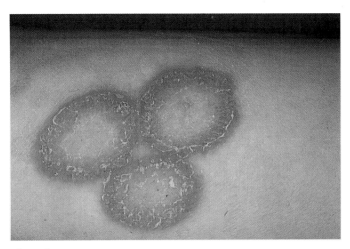

photo 2

TINEA FACIEI

The dermatophytosis has the same appearance as on glabrous skin, but can assume an impressive clinical picture owing to its spread (photo 1) or a more or less atypical one (photo 2) owing to late diagnosis or unsuitable topical therapy with corticosteroids.

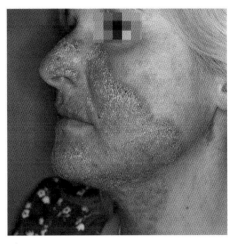

photo 1

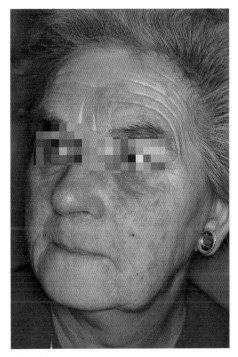

photo 2

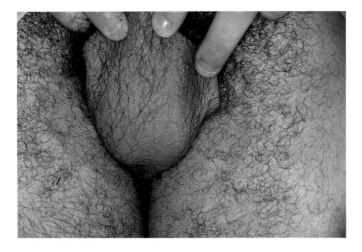

TINEA CRURIS

Dermatophytosis of the inguinal fold (also called dhobi itch and Hebra's eczema marginatum). This dermatophytosis affects men more frequently than women. A very distinct vesicular border circumscribes a central red, sometimes brownish, central region, which is always scaly. The lesion typically spreads towards the inner thigh.

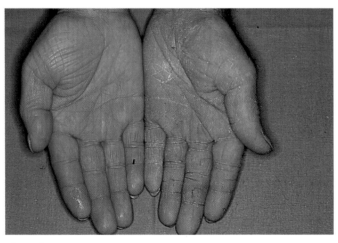

photo 1

TINEA MANUUM

This condition affects the palms, most frequently on one hand (photo 1). It is characterized by diffuse redness and dryness with floury accentuation (photo 2) of flexural creases of the palms .
There is no substantial hyperkeratosis. An active margin may be noticeable at the wrist. Association with athlete's foot or eczema marginatum is typical, and it is a good idea to persevere in looking for this. Scraping with a curette generally yields plenty of horny, brittle, powdery material.

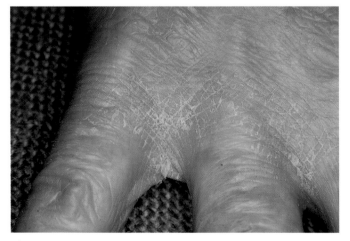

photo 2

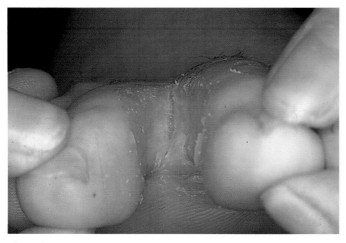

photo 1

TINEA PEDUM (ATHLETE'S FOOT)

Fissured and scaly intertrigo of the space between the fourth and fifth toes. There is often a small painful crack running along the base of the fold (photo 1).
Sometimes the whole area is eroded, which is a sign of microbial infection (photo 2). The dermatophytosis can extend to the sole, which it affects more or less extensively (photo 3).
In some cases in which *tinea manuum* is associated with *tinea pedis*, three of the four limbs are affected (e.g. one hand and two feet).

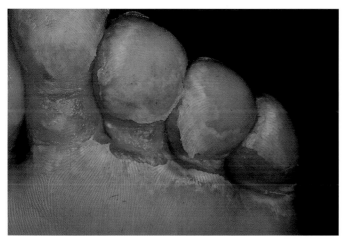

photo 2

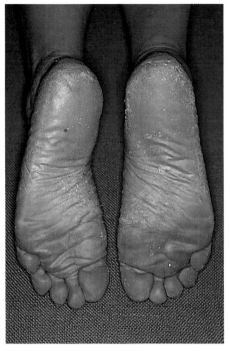

photo 3

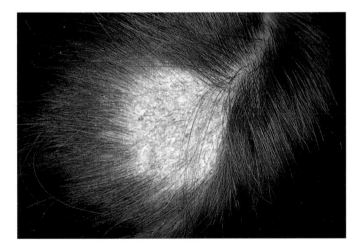

TINEA CAPITIS OR RINGWORM

The scalp is attacked by a dermatophyte. Children are affected most often. Large plaque of alopecia, presence of numerous short broken hairs on a greyish and scaly base. The pathogen is most frequently *Microsporum canis*. Ringworm is characteristic of the prepubescent period: it is distinguished from alopecia or pseudo-alopecia by its floury appearance.

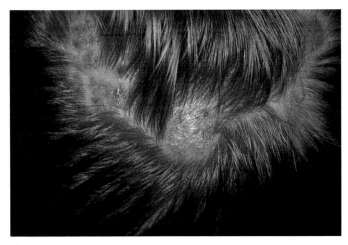

KERION

Crusty and well demarcated suppurative patch, sometimes tumour-like. The most typical site is the scalp in the child (photo 1) and the beard in the adult (photo 2). The lesion evolves into a definitive scar (photo 3). The pathogen is *Trichophyton mentagrophytes* or *Trichophyton verrucosum*.

photo 1

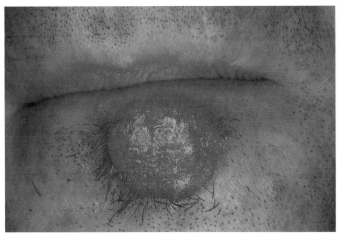

photo 2

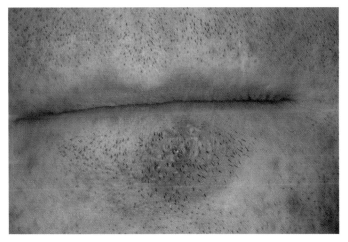

photo 3

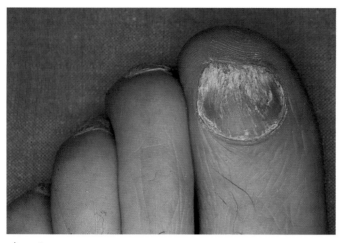

photo 1

ONYCHOMYCOSIS DUE TO DERMATOPHYTES

Thickened and opaque nail, distal onycholysis. The nail becomes brittle. There is no associated paronychia (photo 1). More rarely, dermatophytic onychomycosis involves the superficial layer of the nail plate and appears in the form of small opaque whitish patches which are well demarcated (appearance of leuconychia; photo 2). The surface becomes more brittle as a result.

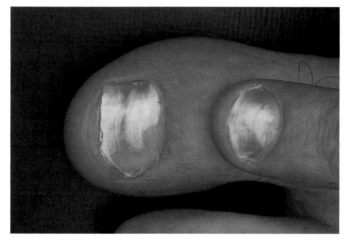

photo 2

CANDIDIASIS

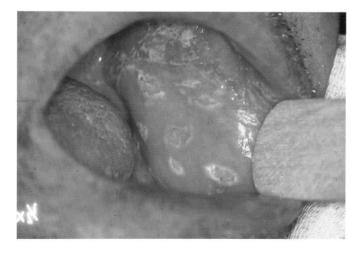

THRUSH

Thrush is the classical form of intraoral candidiasis, characterized by a whitish coating of creamy consistency covering bright red areas of erosion. Scraping with the curette removes the coating and exposes the erosion patches. The inner cheek surface and the tongue are affected. The surrounding mucosa is inflamed and there is a considerable burning sensation. The pathogen is *Candida albicans*.

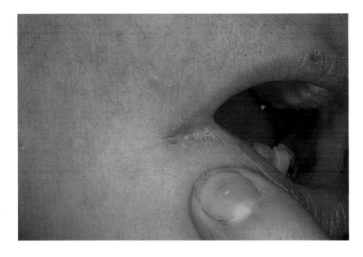

ANGULAR CHEILITIS
Fissures, which are most frequently symmetrical, localized at the corners of the lips and surrounded by small impetigo-like crusts. Edentulous patients or patients with badly fitting dentures are most frequently affected. A superimposed bacterial infection is very common.

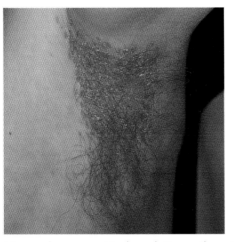

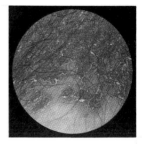

CANDIDAL INTERTRIGO
More or less symmetrical exudative erythematous axillary patches with small satellite lesions. A peripheral desquamative collarette is often present.

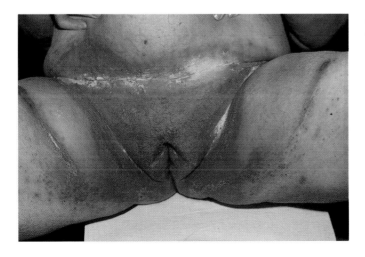

CANDIDAL VULVOVAGINITIS
Symmetrical involvement of the external genitals with peripheral desquamative collarette and small punctiform erythematous satellite lesions which are sometimes somewhat pustular. Itching is generally severe. There is frequently an associated whitish leucorrhoea.

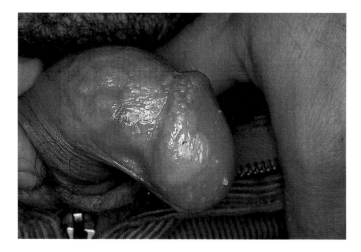

CANDIDAL BALANITIS

Glazed erythema surrounded by a fine whitish border, affecting the glans and the neck of the penis. Relatively intense burning. Recurrences are common.

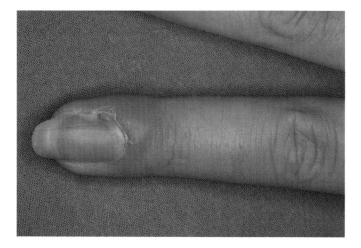

CANDIDAL PARONYCHIA AND SUBUNGUAL INFECTION

Thickened, brittle, and yellowish nail, accompanied by an inflamed nail fold which discharges a purulent exudate on pressure. Pain is typical. Some cases of candidal paronychia are preceded by irritant dermatitis, most frequently to vegetable or animal proteins (protein contact dermatitis).

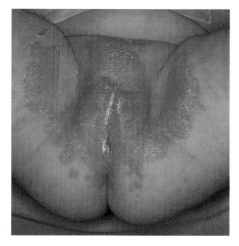

NAPKIN CANDIDIASIS (INFANT)

Wide glazed erythematous patch over the whole area of genitals and buttocks with satellite lesions. The condition classically starts at the base of the folds (inguinal folds, cleft of the buttocks or anal region).

PITYRIASIS VERSICOLOR

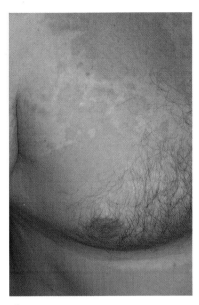

Small, well-demarcated buff or brownish patches located mainly on the trunk or the neck (photo 1). Pruritus is moderate or absent. Scraping with a curette reveals a scale becoming detached from a mass of scales: chip sign (photo 2).

The depigmented form can either be scaly from the beginning and thus contagious, or residual after exposure of pigmented pityriasis versicolor to the sun. In this case it is not contagious and represents only the aftermath of an old pityriasis versicolor after treatment (photo 3). In cases of doubt, mycological examination reveals the presence of short mycelial filaments accompanied by colonies of small round spores *(Malassezia furfur)*. Wood's light examination reveals the presence of a yellowish fluorescence.

photo 1

photo 2

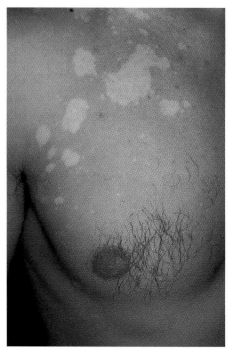

PITYRIASIS VERSICOLOR (continued)

photo 3

DEEP FUNGAL INFECTIONS

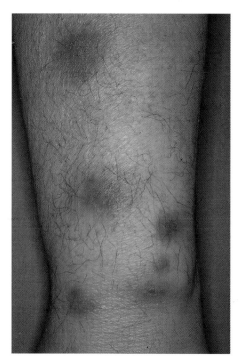

SPOROTRICHOSIS

Multiple violet papulonodular lesions developing along the lines of lymphatic drainage, associated with infection with *Sporothrix schenkii*. The limbs are most frequently affected.

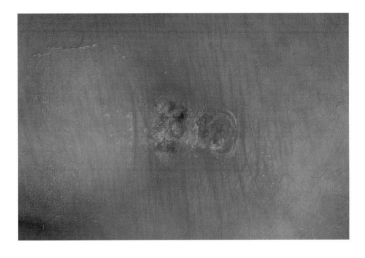

MYCETOMA (MADURA FOOT)

Severe inflammatory swelling located most frequently on the foot, exuding a purulent material containing grains through fine breaks. The pathogens can be either eumycetes or actinomycetes.

E. Parasitic diseases - Arthropods

HUMAN SCABIES

Parasitic disease caused by *Sarcoptes scabiei*. Blackish burrows from 5 to 15 mm in length, ending in a vesicle at one end ("mite hill"). The sides of the fingers and the anterior surfaces of the wrist are sites of predilection (photo 1). Numerous marks of excoriation, sometimes accompanied by fine more or less translucent vesicles spread all over the skin. These excoriations are mainly the sign of very severe itching in the evening and at night (photo 2). Scabies nodules: very distinctly infiltrated, extremely itchy reddish nodules in the axillae, on the scrotum, and on the penis, persisting even after successful treatment (photo 3).
In children the lesions usually affect the feet: numerous extremely itchy excoriated papules (photo 4).

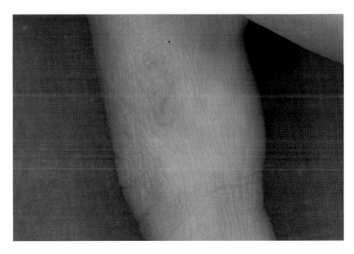

photo 1

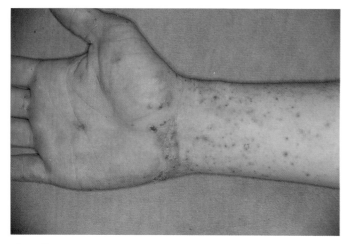

photo 2

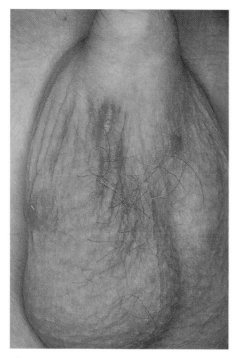

photo 3

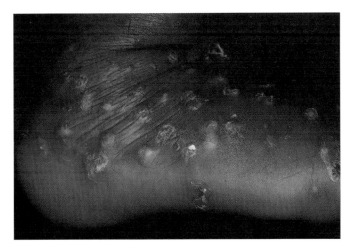

photo 4

ANIMAL SCABIES

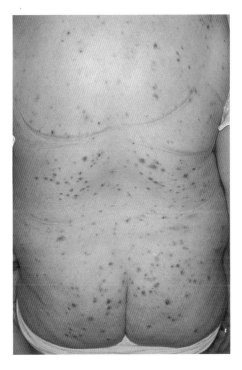

Numerous small itchy papules spread all over the skin, which regress spontaneously. There are no burrows. The patient's pet (cat or dog) is typically found to be infested.

PEDICULOSIS (HEAD LICE)

Wide impetigo-like patch at the nape of the neck caused by scratching, associated with very severe undiagnosed infestation (photo 1). Area of attachment of a nit to a hair (photo 2).

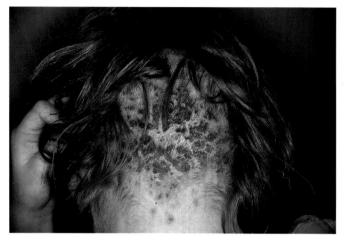

photo 1

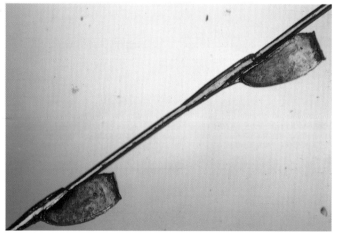

photo 2

CRAB LICE (PUBIC LICE)

Excoriations and presence of louse eggs firmly attached to the pubic hairs. There are also crab lice *(Phthirius pubis)* grasping the pubic hairs (photo 1). On the body, relatively discrete bluish grey macules *(maculae caerulae)* can sometimes be found. These blue-grey macules correspond to the release of toxins by the crab louse in the course of successive bites (photo 2).

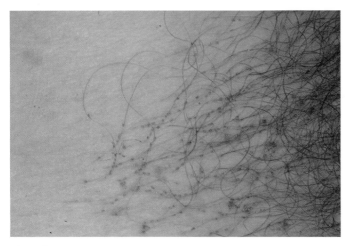

photo 1

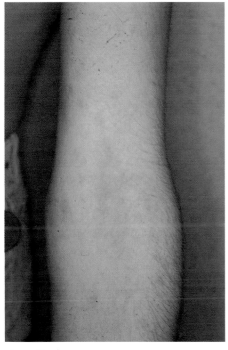

photo 2

INSECT BITES

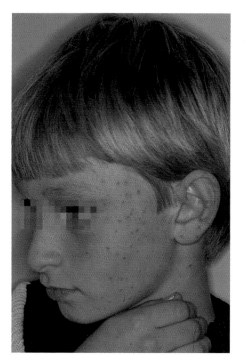

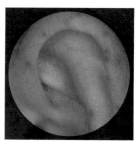

TROMBICULIASIS

Immunological reactions to bites by harvest mites (*larvae* of *Trombiculidae* which feed on blood). Small itchy lesions, sometimes in a line, located anywhere on the skin, with predilection for constricted areas. The lesions sometimes rise to a point in the centre.

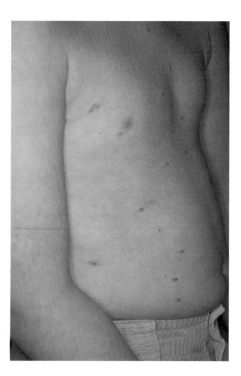

INFANTILE PAPULAR URTICARIA (STROPHULUS)

Occuring mainly in children, this type of papular urticaria occurs in the form of numerous small erythematous papules, sometimes with fine vesicles. The lesions are found mainly on the legs, are extremely itchy, and very likely to be excoriated. Sometimes a linear disposition is seen, which makes the diagnosis much more obvious. Infantile papular urticaria is caused by an ectoparasite with a cat or dog host.

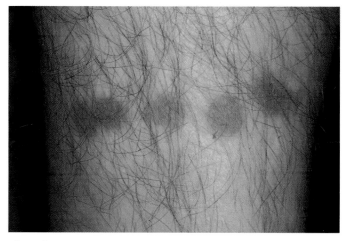

FLEA BITES

Large inflammatory papules in a linear disposition. There is a distinct central acumination. Infestation is usually via a pet (cat or dog), which acts as the carrier (photo 1). In some cases the lesions become frankly bullous and even haemorrhagic (photo 2).

photo 1

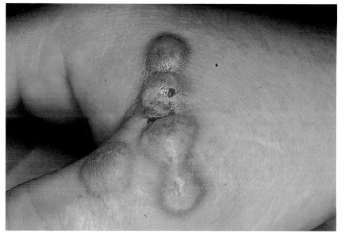

photo 2

LEISHMANIASIS

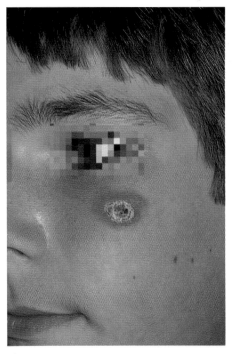

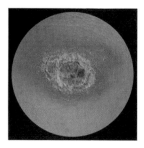

Large encrusted papular lesion surrounded by an inflammatory rim. There is no associated pain or lymphadenopathy. The course is chronic and the lesion is resistant to conventional antiseptic treatments (photo 1). After a few months the lesion subsides, leaving a scar of variable visibility (photo 2). It is a protozoan infection caused by a species of Leishmania. The carrier is a Phlebotomus fly, which explains why in most cases the lesions of leishmaniasis are found on uncovered areas (especially the face).

photo 1

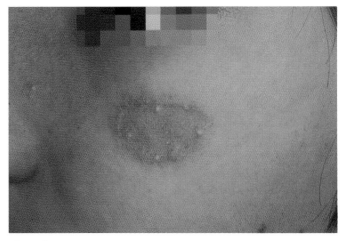

photo 2

LARVA MIGRANS (CREEPING ERUPTION)

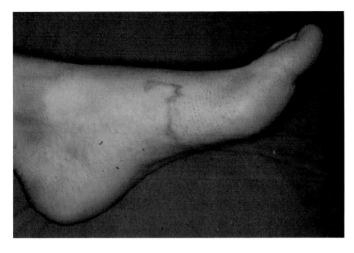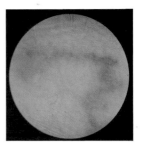

Inflammatory serpiginous line ending in a small, extremely itchy papule. *Larva migrans* is caused by a larva of an Ancylostoma species (hookworm) which migrates about 1 cm per day, thus extending the line of inflammation. In humans contact usually occurs on the beach (soil polluted with animal excreta).
Cutaneous *larva migrans* is found mainly on the feet and the buttocks.

TUNGIASIS (CHIGGER)

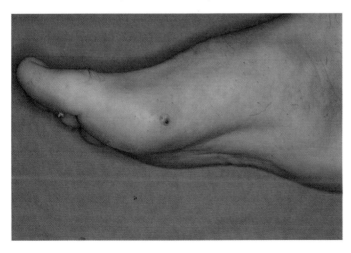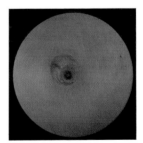

Itchy inflammatory nodule with a small blackish opening at the centre, found in the periungual region of a toe. Secondary superinfection (abscess formation) may be present. Tungiasis is caused by a flea which lives on blood: *Tunga penetrans*. Infestation typically occurs on the feet (walking barefoot in areas where it is endemic, especially Africa and Central America).

PSORIASIS

CLINICAL ASPECTS

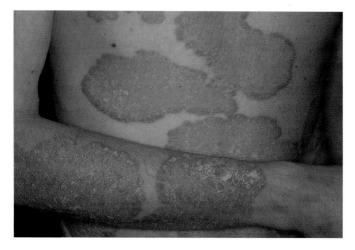

PSORIASIS VULGARIS
Erythematous form
Very extensive psoriasis.
Large confluent patches,
mainly erythematous,
covered in fine scales.

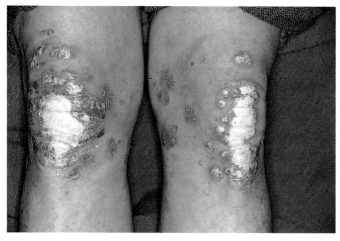

Scaly erythematous form
Psoriasis on the knees. Well-demarcated scaly erythematous patches. Thick white scales with a shiny micaceous appearance.

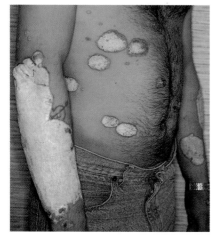

Plaster-like psoriasis
Extended psoriatic lesions on the trunk and the arms. In the present case the scales, which are thick and adherent, mask the erythema which appears here and there like a thin border at the edge of the lesions. The appearance of the scales is such that they are often referred to as cretaceous psoriasis or, more picturesquely, "plaster-like scales".

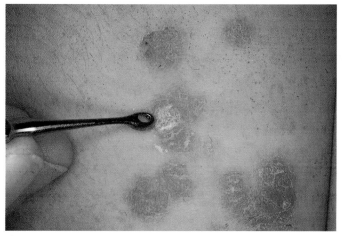

photo 1

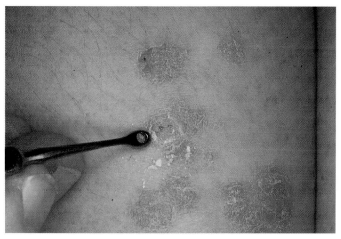

photo 2

Characteristic clinical symptoms
Patches resemble candle wax (photo 1) and are bleeding (photo 2) after curettage.

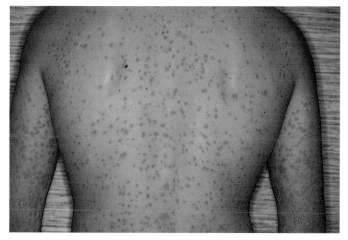

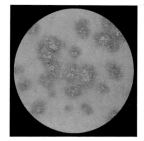

Guttate psoriasis

Guttate psoriasis consists of innumerable small scaly erythematous patches, a few millimetres across, which in the present case are distributed all over the skin. In many cases it is an eruptive psoriasis of childhood or adolescence.

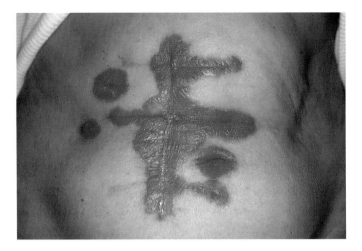

Kœbner's phenomenon
(isomorphic reaction).
Psoriatic lesions appear
around a surgical scar.

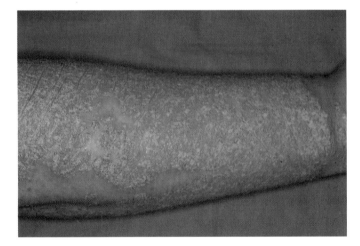

PUSTULAR PSORIASIS
Body
Pustular psoriasis of the
flexor surface of the forearm.
Large erythematous patch
with distinct margins, strewn
with a scatter of flattened
yellowish-white pustules
arranged in confluent
clusters.

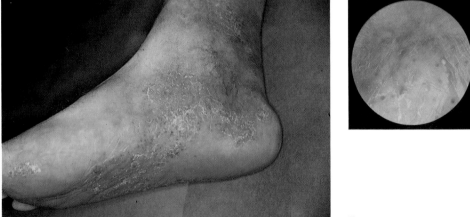

Feet

Plantar pustular psoriasis. Isolated pustules appear on a scaly erythematous base with distinct borders. The most recent yellowish-white pustules are slightly raised, whereas the older pustules are brown and embedded in the horny layer of the epidermis.

PSORIATIC ERYTHRODERMA

Psoriatic erythroderma. The erythrodermic psoriasis has spread all over the body (photo 1) without intervals of healthy skin (photo 2).

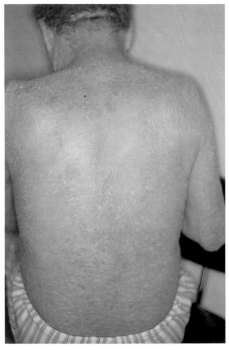

photo 1

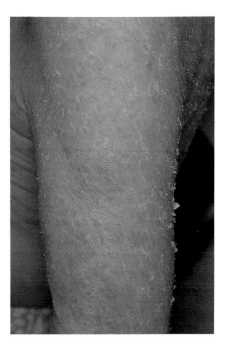

photo 2

PARTICULAR LOCAL FORMS

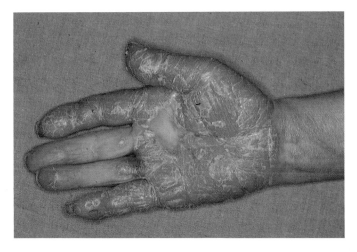

PALMOPLANTAR PSORIASIS

Palmar psoriasis. Scaly erythematous patches with distinctly rounded contours. The covering scales are thick and nacreous.

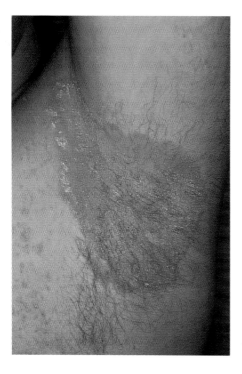

FLEXURAL PSORIASIS
Inverse psoriasis of an axilla. The psoriatic eruption consists of a continuous plaque which is bright red, shiny, smooth, and not very scaly, with a well-circumscribed margin.

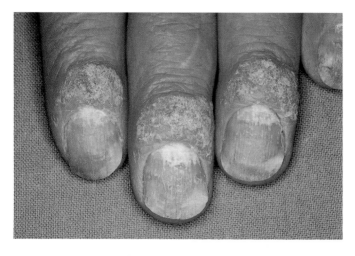

PSORIASIS OF THE NAILS
The picture, which is very complete, includes distal onycholysis with yellow coloration, cup-shaped depressions in the central area, and advanced disintegration of the nail plate in the proximal area. In addition, classical psoriatic lesions have invaded the whole of the nail fold.

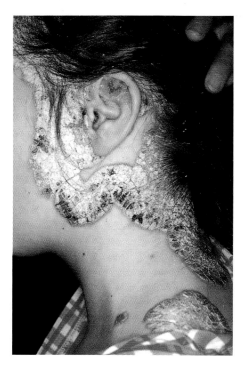

PSORIASIS OF THE SCALP
The round, scaly erythematous patches spread beyond the hairline to invade the cervical region.

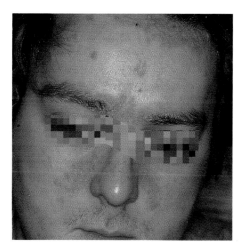

PSORIASIS OF THE FACE (SEBORRHOEIC PSORIASIS)
Psoriasis of the face is rare and is usually found predominantly in the seborrhoeic regions: wings of the nose, area between the eyebrows, hairline. It is often called "seborrhoeic psoriasis".

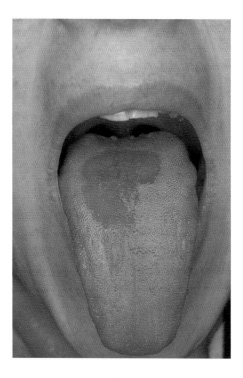

MUCOSAL PSORIASIS
1. Psoriasis of the tongue
Erythematous and slightly glazed plaques with distinct margins, scattered over the upper surface of the tongue.

The picture is quite similar to that described by the term geographical tongue (or benign migratory glossitis or lingual *erythema migrans*).

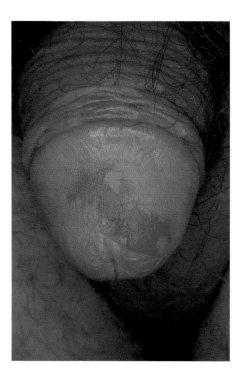

2. Psoriasis of the glans penis
Large red and well-circumscribed plaques, neither infiltrated nor scaly, with a chronic course. They present problems of differential diagnosis, as they have to be distinguished from balanitis of other origins.

OTHER SKIN DISEASES

PITYRIASIS ROSEA

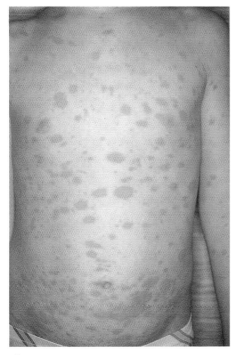

The eruption consists of pink oval patches measuring 1 to 3 cm in diameter, with fine scaling in a peripheral collarette (photo 1).
The initial lesion, looking like an oval medallion, can usually be recognized by its larger size (diameter 5 to 6 cm) and its accentuated margin. Its oblique orientation on the trunk is characteristic (photo 2).

photo 1

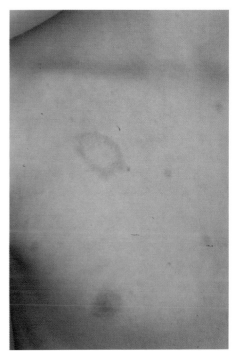

photo 2

PARAPSORIASIS

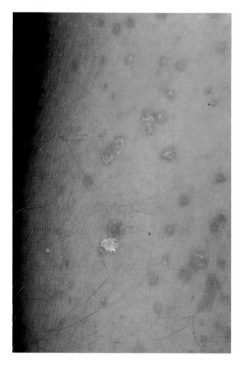

PITYRIASIS LICHENOIDES ("GUTTATE PARAPSORIASIS")

The polymorphic eruption is spread over the trunk and the limbs. It consists of red or brownish and more or less scaly maculopapular lesions.
The characteristic feature is a brownish macule covered with an adherent scale, which detaches in one piece.

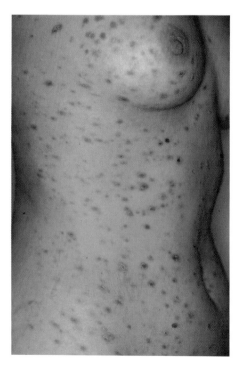

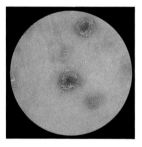

VARIOLOID PARAPSORIASIS

The eruption affects the trunk and the limbs. It is polymorphic: papulopustular lesions, necrotic, often haemorrhagic lesions, crusts, varioloid scars.

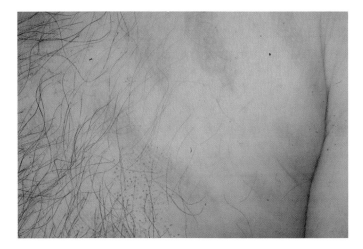

CHRONIC SUPERFICIAL SCALY DERMATITIS (DIGITATE DERMATOSIS)

The lesions are oval, 2 to 5 cm in diameter, well-circumscribed, flat, and yellowish pink with fine scaling. These patches are disposed in lines, the position of which is fairly stereotyped: slanting along the ribs on the trunk, longitudinal on the limbs.

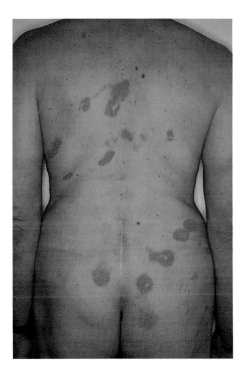

PREMYCOTIC OR PRERETICULOTIC ERUPTION WITH LARGE PLAQUES

The lesions consist of wide plaques (10 to 20 cm in diameter) located on the trunk and the base of the limbs. Their appearance is polymorphic: sepia-coloured scaly erythematous plaques, atrophic or even poikilodermal lesions.

LICHEN PLANUS

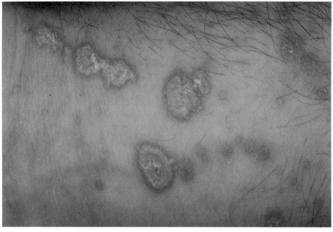

photo 1

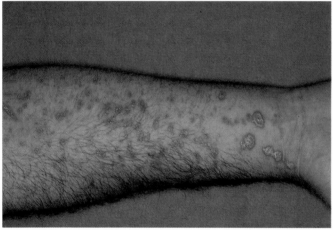

photo 2

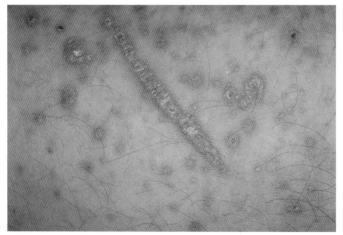

photo 3

SIMPLE CUTANEOUS LICHEN PLANUS

The basic lesion is a firm reddish-violet polygon. The surface, which has a sheen in oblique illumination, is covered with fine greyish striations known as Wickham's striae (photo 1).

One of the preferred sites is the flexor surface of the forearm (photo 2).

Papules may appear along the excoriations caused by scratching (Kœbner's phenomenon; photo 3).

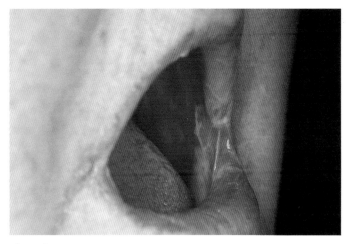

photo 1

ORAL LICHEN PLANUS

The lesions are white and reticulated. Their preferred site is the tongue and the lower posterior part of the cheeks ("fern-leaf" appearance; photo 1).
A rare form is erosive lichen planus: painful red ulcerations with no tendency towards spontaneous healing (photo 2). The ulcers are surrounded by a lichen-like whitish border.

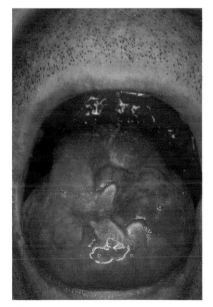

photo 2

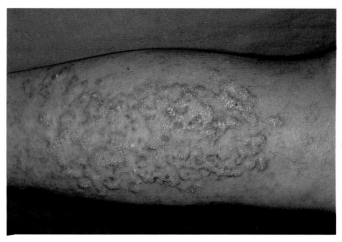

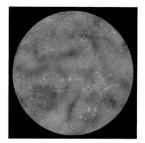

HYPERTROPHIC
LICHEN PLANUS

The lesions are oval or coalescent, infiltrated, and pink or violet in colour.
Their surface is hyperkeratotic. This skin disease classically affects the front of the legs.

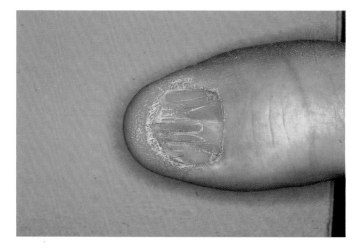

LICHEN PLANUS OF
THE NAILS

Dorsal pterygium and flaps
of nail at the sides.

GRAFT VERSUS HOST DISEASE (GVHD)

In the subacute stage the graft's reaction against the host can appear as a lichenoid eruption. The lesions are spread all over the skin (photo 1) and can involve the mucosa (photo 2).

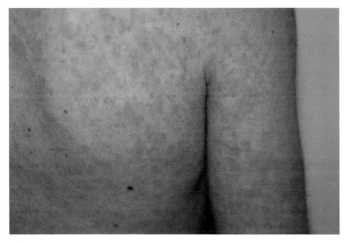

photo 1

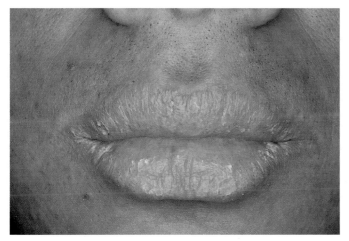

photo 2

LICHENIFICATION

Well-demarcated thick itchy hyperkeratotic patch on the ankle, forming a grid of scratch lines. The term neurodermatitis is sometimes used to describe this phenomenon.

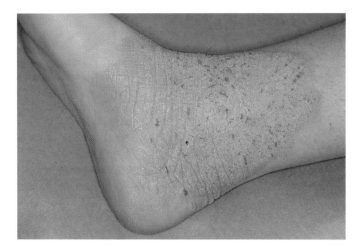

SUBACUTE PRURIGO

The excoriated papules are disposed symmetrically on the extensor surfaces of the limbs (photo 1), the upper back (photo 2), and sometimes on the face and the scalp.

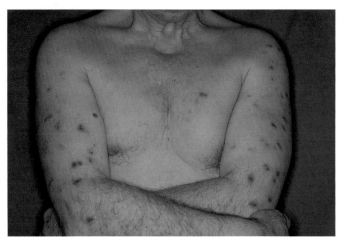

photo 1

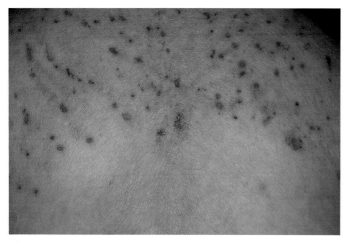

photo 2

LUPUS ERYTHEMATOSUS

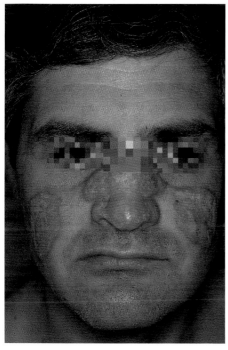

photo 1

DISCOID LUPUS ERYTHEMATOSUS
1. Face

The eruption consists of erythematous patches covered with an adherent hyperkeratotic layer, predominantly at the hair follicles. It resolves into cicatricial atrophy (photo 1).

A rare form is lupus erythematosus tumidus. The erythema is associated with severe oedema, producing one or more swollen patches with distinct margins, a smooth surface, and an oedematous consistency (photo 2).

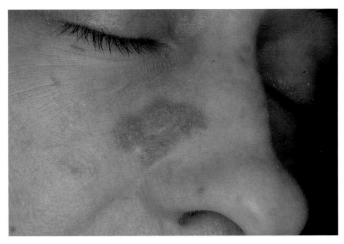

DISCOID LUPUS ERYTHEMATOSUS (continued)

photo 2

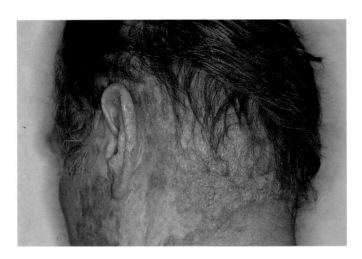

2. Scalp
This consists of erythematous and somewhat atrophic alopecic plaques which heal with scarring.

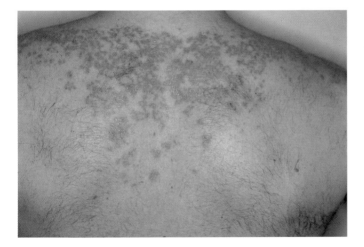

SUBACUTE LUPUS ERYTHEMATOSUS
The eruption corresponds to a profuse form consisting of erythematous and somewhat scaly polycyclic annular plaques which resolve to leave depigmentation and telangiectasia.

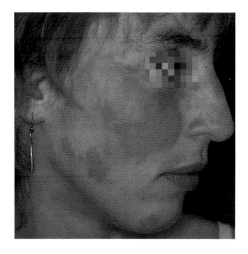

SYSTEMIC LUPUS ERYTHEMATOSUS
1. Face
The eruption is in the form of slightly oedematous erythematous sheets, without atrophy or follicular hyperkeratosis.

The lesions are often symmetrical and located on areas exposed to the sun ("butterfly" appearance).

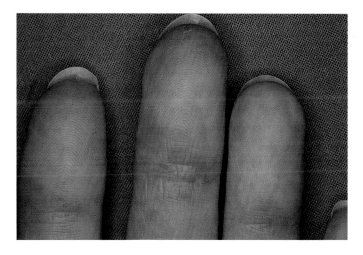

2. Fingers
The site of the lesions on the fingers is usually around the nails. The lesions are usually erythematous and telangiectatic, sometimes violet (chilblain-like in appearance).

JESSNER AND KANOF DISEASE

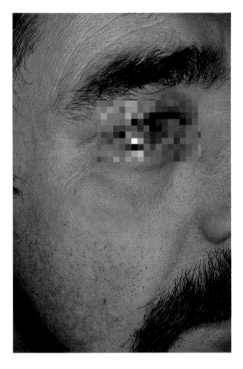

The eruption consists of more or less tumid smooth erythematous papules with a flat surface and no scaling. These lesions tend to be located on the face, neck, and the upper trunk.

DERMATOMYOSITIS

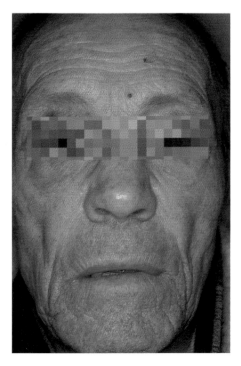

1. Face
Diffuse oedematous and telangiectatic erythema of the face. The lesions are usually found predominantly on the eyelids.

2. Hands and fingers

Lesions of purplish erythema predominantly on the dorsal surface of the hand and finger joints, mainly in the supra-articular regions.

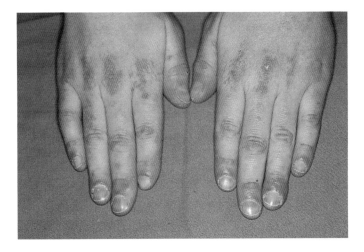

SCLERODERMA

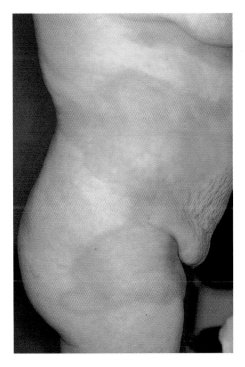

LOCALIZED MORPHOEA
1. Plaque lesions

The condition consists of one or more indurated nacreous white plaques which have a sheen in oblique light. They are bordered by a mauve band (lilac ring) which disappears as the lesions develop.

2. Bands

This variant of morphoea is characterized by a paramedian band of sclerosis and atrophy. In some cases actual facial hemiatrophy develops.

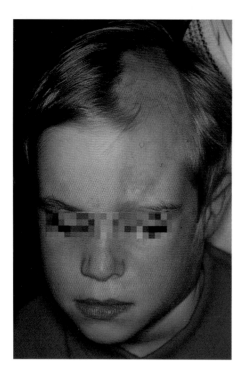

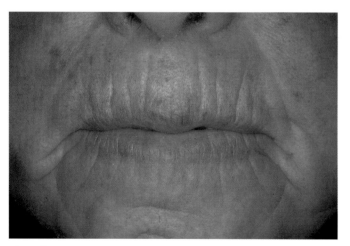

photo 1

SYSTEMIC SCLEROSIS

Systemic sclerosis is found mainly on the face and on the extremities. The facial expression seems fixed. The tapering of the nose and narrowing of the mouth, surrounded by radial furrows, aggravate the lack of expression (photo 1). The sclerodactyly is characterized by tapering of the fingers, which become fixed in flexion (photo 2). There are painful ulcerations on the pulps.

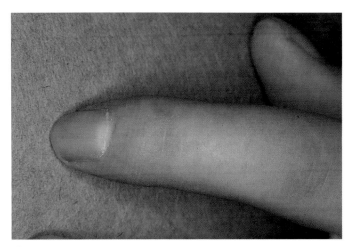

photo 2

LICHEN SCLEROSUS

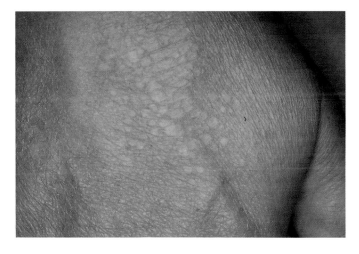

SKIN (GLABROUS SKIN)
Well-circumscribed shiny white papules resembling mother-of-pearl, with a slight depression at the centre, sometimes clustered in plaques with fragmented margins.

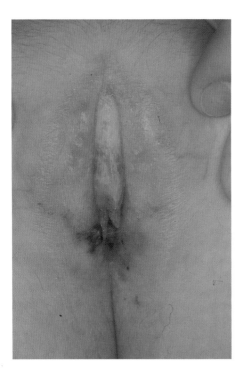

VULVA
The vulval mucosa assumes a nacreous white shiny appearance. There are sometimes areas of bruising.

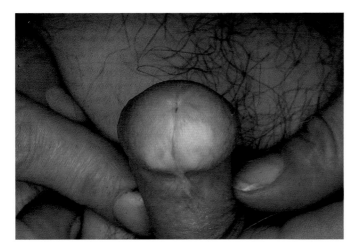

GLANS PENIS
Porcelain-white patches which are either disseminated or, more often, located around the meatus.

SARCOIDOSIS

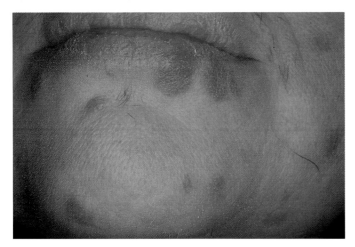

PAPULAR FORM
Small, round, well-circumscribed elevations, either isolated or multiple, measuring 1 to 3 mm in diameter. Their colour is red, violet, or sepia. They appear yellowish on vitropression.

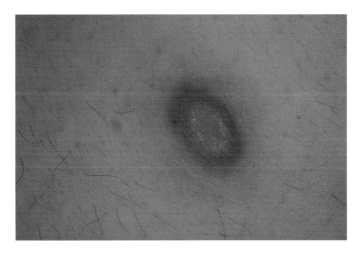

NODULAR FORM
Larger lesions (diameter 5 to 10 mm). These are smooth, firm, violet or brownish red, and have the same appearance of yellowish lupoid infiltration on vitropression.

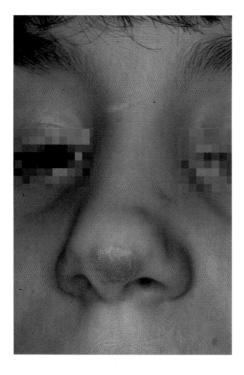

ANGIOLUPOID FORM
This very rare clinical variant consists of a tumid, round or oval, reddish violet infiltration appearing on the nose.

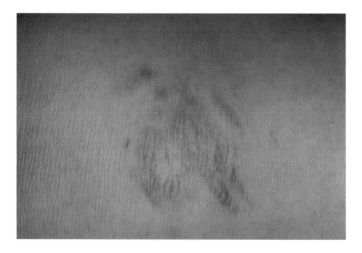

SCAR SARCOIDOSIS
Development of sarcoid nodules around foreign matter contained in a scar. These nodules sometimes appear in the context of active systemic sarcoidosis. Sometimes, however, they represent a simple local granulomatous reaction.

GRANULOMA ANNULARE

Small, firm, well-circumscribed nodules with a smooth surface, which are normal or pink in colour and show little inflammation. They are clustered in rings which spread outwards from the centre. The ring does not generally exceed a diameter of 1 to 2 cm. Giant annular granulomas (several centimetres in diameter) are much more rare.

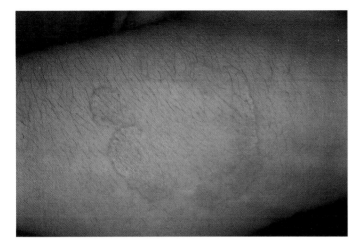

NECROBIOSIS LIPOIDICA

Large sclerotic and atrophic pretibial plaque with distinct margins, red and telangiectatic.
Its surface is shiny, which explains the "hot spot" on the photograph (photo 1).
The centre of the plaque is smooth, with a cicatricial appearance which is often yellowish owing to an excess of fat (photo 2).

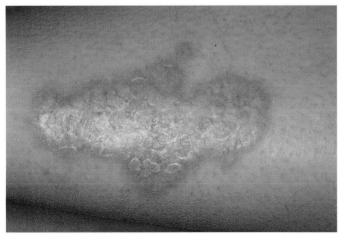

photo 1

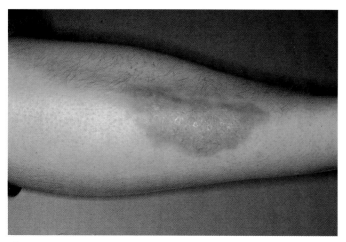

photo 2

VASCULITIS

The term vasculitis is used collectively for diseases associated with inflammation of the walls of blood vessels in the skin and other organs. The classification of vasculitis is usually based on two features: the calibre of the affected vessels and the type of inflammatory reaction. Urticarial vasculitis is included in the section on urticaria.

CUTANEOUS VASCULITIS (ALLERGIC VASCULITIS)

Histologically, cutaneous vasculitis is characterized by infiltration of polymorphonuclear neutrophils, which are often pyknotic, into and around the vessel walls, hence the often-used term leucocytoclastic vasculitis. It occurs in two main well-defined forms: purpuric and necrotic.

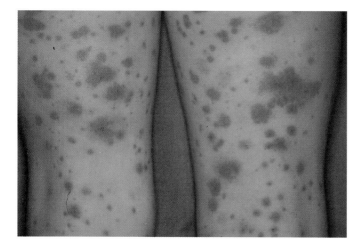

Purpuric form
In this form the lesions essentially correspond to infiltrated purpuric papules, which affect mainly the legs and which can extend over other skin areas.

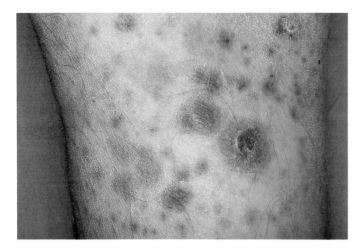

Necrotic form

Purpuric papules coexist with vesiculobullous, pustular, or necrotic lesions, hence the old name used in the French literature: "Gougerot's triad".

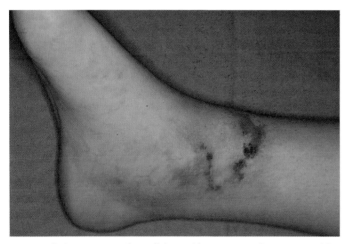

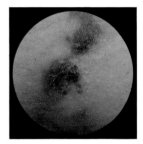

ATROPHIE BLANCHE (LIVEDO VASCULITIS)

Picture of chronic vasculitis of the ankle regions, characterized by purpura which necroses rapidly, leaving very small painful ulcerations bordered by a violet ring.

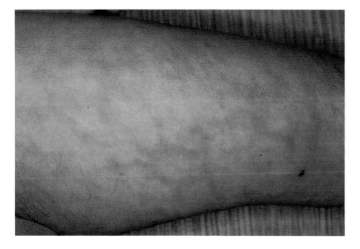

POLYARTERITIS NODOSA

The clinical appearance is generally polymorphic, combining cutaneous nodules, livedo, infiltrated purpura, and necrotic ulcerations. These cutaneous signs are part of general systemic illness (weight loss, fever, aching all over the body).

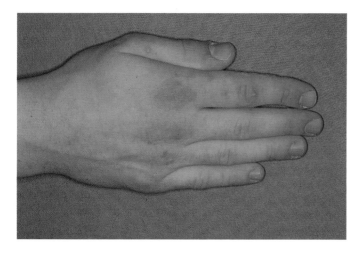

ERYTHEMA ELEVATUM DIUTINUM

Very rare vasculitis characterized by the appearance of red or violet papules, plaques, and nodules distributed symmetrically over the extensor surfaces of the limbs. The course is chronic and successive episodes are accompanied by fever.

ERYTHEMA NODOSUM

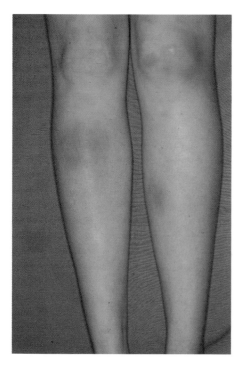

The eruption

Painful red nodules found mainly on the extensor surfaces of the legs, usually accompanied by fever and pains in the joints.

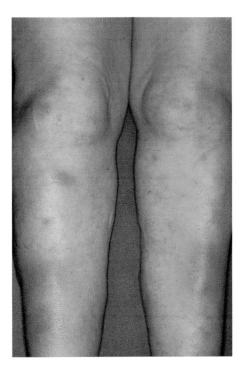

Regression
The nodules resolve in about ten days and turn blue and yellow, like bruises.

NODULAR VASCULITIS (PANNICULITIS)

Firm cyanotic nodules with little inflammation, located on the lower third of the legs. They occur in women, usually overweight women suffering from chronic venous insufficiency.

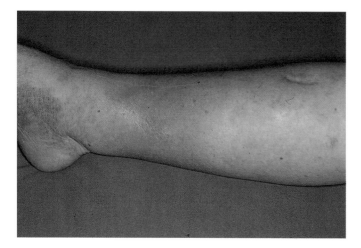

PYODERMA GANGRENOSUM

Superficial ulceration with circular margins, bordered by a firm inflammatory swelling, which is undermined by deep-seated purulent lesions. The condition can be idiopathic or associated with various internal diseases, in particular, diseases of the digestive tract such as Crohn's disease or ulcerative colitis. The illustrations correspond to two stages of development of the same lesion in a leg.

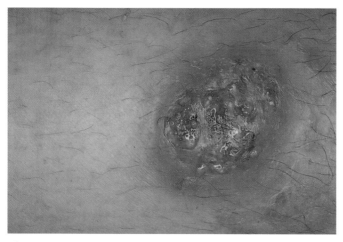

photo 1

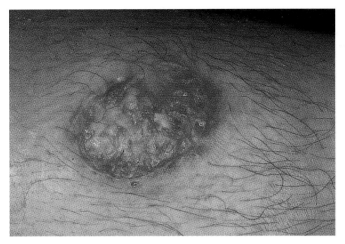

photo 2

ERYTHEMA MULTIFORME

Erythema multiforme is a syndrome of the skin and mucosa associated with various aetiological circumstances, among which herpes infections occupy an important place.

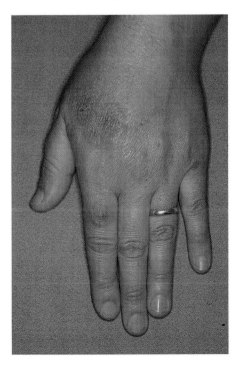

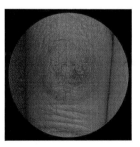

Non-bullous "target" form

Dull red, round, symmetrical maculopapules on the backs of the hands. The characteristic configuration is like a target or butterfly.

Bullous form

The maculopapules in a butterfly configuration are bullous in the centre and can follow a necrotic course. The mucous membranes are sometimes affected.

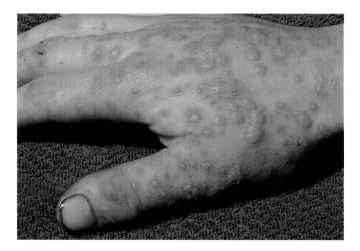

Stevens-Johnson syndrome

This is the most severe form of erythema multiforme. In addition to the cutaneous symptoms there are severe erosive mucosal lesions affecting the lips, buccal cavity, and sometimes the genital organs. The clinical picture is severe, with fever and alterations of the general condition.

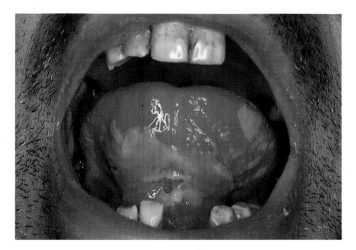

SWEET'S SYNDROME (ACUTE FEBRILE NEUTROPHILIC DERMATOSIS)

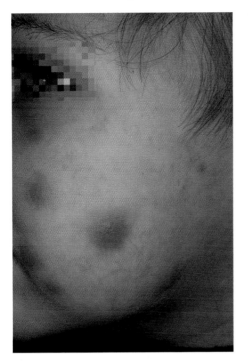

Well-circumscribed infiltrated erythematous plaques, depressed at the centre, appearing on the limbs. Raised temperature, aching joints, abdominal pain, and neutrophilia accompany the skin symptoms.

BULLOUS PEMPHIGOID

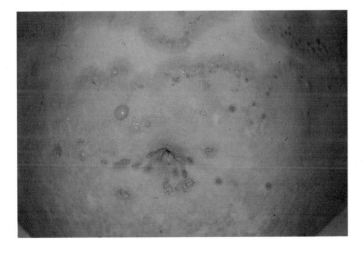

Early stage
Large urticaria-like polycyclic patches, bordered by a few firm bullae of varying size and containing a clear liquid.

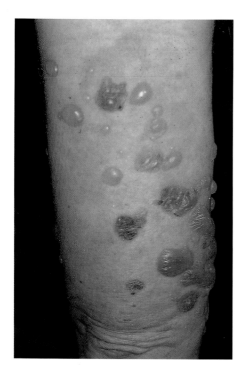

Further development
Presence of very numerous firm bullae of varying size, some of which are haemorrhagic. Some bullae rupture, leaving extensive skin erosions.

AUTOIMMUNE FORMS OF PEMPHIGUS

Two forms of autoimmune pemphigus are distinguished, according to the preferred site of separation of epidermal cells from each other: "**deep**" pemphigus (*pemphigus vulgaris* and *pemphigus vegetans*) on the one hand and "**superficial**" pemphigus (*pemphigus erythematosus*) on the other.

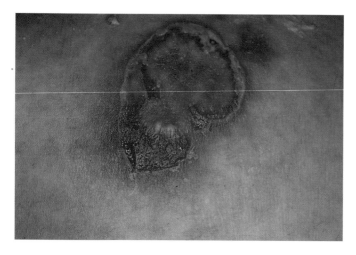

PEMPHIGUS VULGARIS
Skin
Presence of superficial flaccid bullae, which rupture easily to expose extensive erosions.

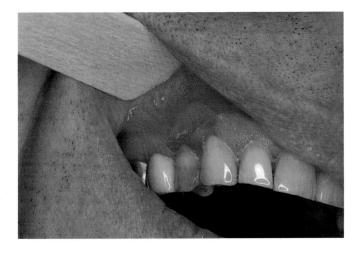

Oral

Dragging painful erosions of the buccal mucosa of the inside of the cheeks, the palate, and the dental cuffs, exposing a bright red surface without a fibrinous coating. Similar erosions can occur in other bullous diseases, but in pemphigus they are more constant and more characteristic.

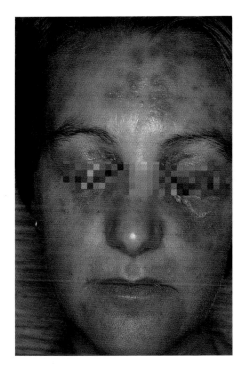

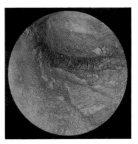

PEMPHIGUS ERYTHEMATOSUS

Crusty, scaly, erythematous plaques of the seborrhoeic regions on the face and the trunk, which are sometimes itchy. These lesions represent the development of superficial bullae.
This variant is also characteristic of drug-induced pemphigus (d-penicillamine).

BENIGN FAMILIAL CHRONIC PEMPHIGUS (HAILEY-HAILEY DISEASE)

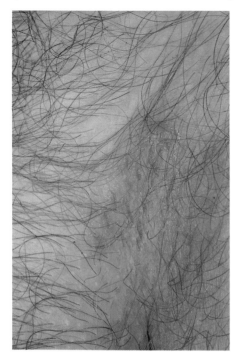

Erosive vesiculobullous lesions which become covered with small yellowish crusts. The lesions are clustered in well-defined plaques traversed by very characteristic parallel fissures. The preferred sites of these lesions are the sides of the neck, the axillae, and the inguinogenital region.

DERMATITIS HERPETIFORMIS

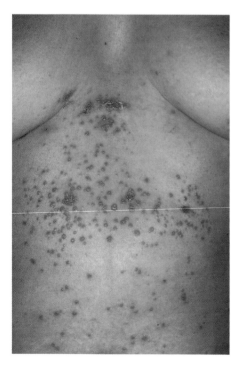

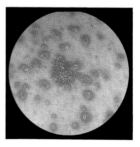

Urticaria-like erythematous or papular lesions surmounted by vesicles and bullae, clustered in a herpetiform ring. The symmetry of the lesions, the constant pruritus, and the association with a gluten-sensitive enteric disease are the other peculiarities of this rare skin disease.

LINEAR IgA BULLOUS DISEASE

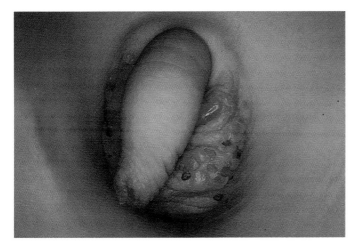

Large firm bullae containing a clear liquid, occurring on normal or erythematous skin. The usual sites are the lower part of the trunk, buttocks, perineum, and the thighs. This chronic bullous skin disease of children and adults is characterized by linear deposits of IgA in direct immunofluorescence.

EPIDERMOLYSIS BULLOSA

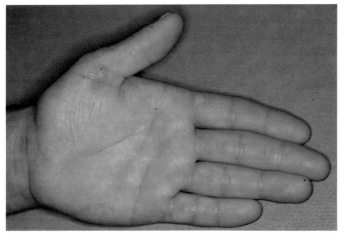

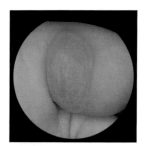

SIMPLE EPIDERMOLYSIS BULLOSA (NON-DYSTROPHIC)

Clear bullae of various sizes, triggered by trauma and by persistent friction, which heal without leaving a trace. The usual sites are the hands, feet, elbows, and knees in the adult and the bottom in the infant. There is no abnormality of the teeth or the nails. The condition is transmitted in the autosomal dominant mode.

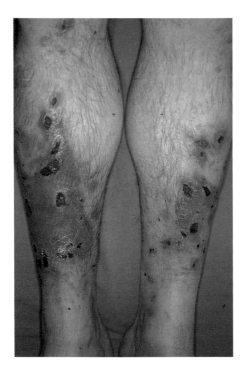

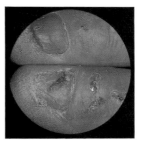

DYSTROPHIC FORMS OF EPIDERMOLYSIS BULLOSA

In dystrophic forms of epidermolysis bullosa, of which there are a number of variants, the traumatic bullae leave atrophic scars and milia when they heal. Some joints can be fixed in flexion. Certain abnormalities of the teeth or the nails are sometimes associated. The mode of transmission varies according to the form of the disease.

DIABETIC BULLAE

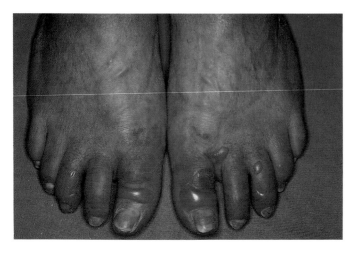

Translucent bullae of various sizes, haemorrhagic in rare cases, without inflammatory areola, which are usually multiple, found especially on the extremities, particularly on the feet. The condition tends to occur in complicated cases of diabetes of all types.

PORPHYRIA CUTANEA TARDA

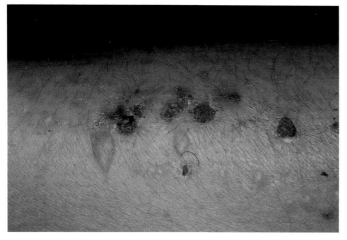

photo 1

The preferred sites of porphyria cutanea tarda lesions are areas exposed to light, such as the backs of the hands and the face. On the backs of the hands the condition is characterized by several symptoms associated with increased skin fragility: serous or haemorrhagic bullae (photo 1), erosions after various traumas, milia (photo 2). On the face the condition is characterized mainly by hypertrichosis of the malar regions and a diffuse brownish pigmentation.

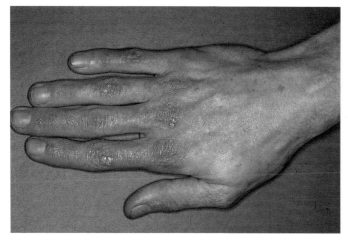

photo 2

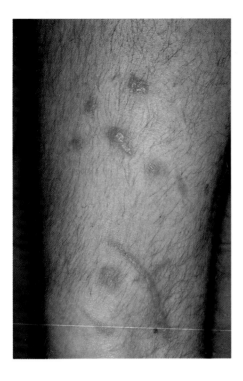

BULLOUS PHYTOPHOTODERMATITIS (MEADOW DERMATITIS)

Erythematous vesicular or bullous eruption reproducing the pattern of a grass or leaf. Sun, humidity, and contact with the plant are the three prerequisites for the appearance of this skin condition.

ACNE AND ROSACEA

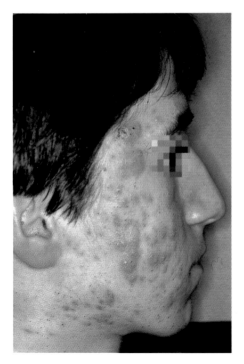

ACNE VULGARIS

Acne vulgaris (adolescent acne) essentially includes three types of lesion: comedones, papules, and pustules. To these can be added nodules and cysts.

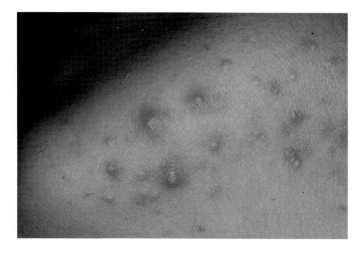

Papulopustular acne
Papulopustular acne essentially comprises isolated or confluent papules and very inflamed papulopustules. It is often associated with seborrhoea. Comedones are never absent.

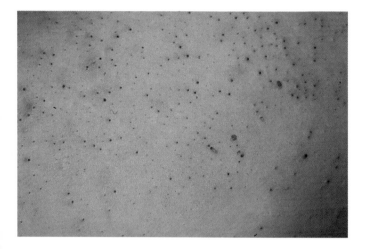

Comedo acne
Comedo acne is characterized by a distinct preponderance of comedones over the lesions of adolescent acne.
The comedones are either open (blackheads) or closed (whiteheads). Blackheads are the prominent lesions in this illustration. Cosmetic acne often takes the form of this variant.

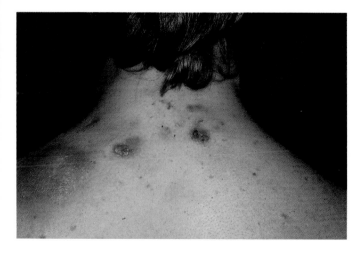

Nodular and cystic acne
In addition to the basic lesions just mentioned (comedones, papules, and pustules), this form of acne presents epidermal cysts of follicular origin and inflamed nodules resulting from the rupture of these cysts.
The nodules can develop into abscesses, which leave indurated, pitted, or retractile scars when they dry out.

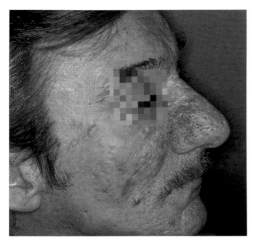
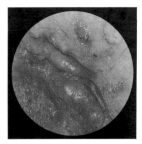

ACNE CONGLOBATA

The lesions are polymorphic and numerous: multiple comedones, follicular cysts, pustules, nodules, and abscesses developing to form fistulae, haemorrhagic ulcers, then pitted scars and adhesions bridging the scars.
This form of acne classically affects the face and trunk, but it can also spread to the arms and the buttocks.

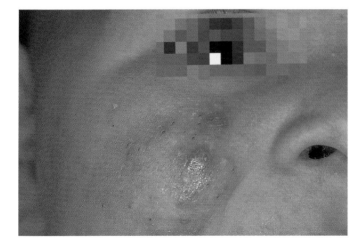

INFANTILE ACNE (ACNE INFANTUM)

This variant of acne, of indeterminate origin, appears in infants aged between 3 and 6 months. It is usually severe, but in most cases fades in 1 to 2 years. It is characterized by the presence of comedones, papules, and pustules, found mainly on the cheeks.
It should be distinguished from a much more rare variety of acne: neonatal acne (acne neonatorum).

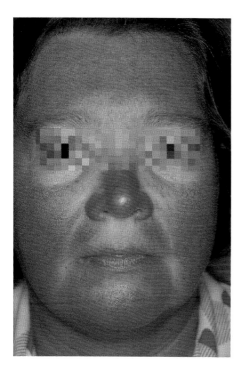

ROSACEA
Blotchy form
The blotchy form comprises erythema and telangiectasia affecting the nose, cheeks, and sometimes the forehead and chin. Flushes appear in various circumstances: in the presence of stress or a change in ambient temperature, after the consumption of alcohol, hot drinks, or hot food.

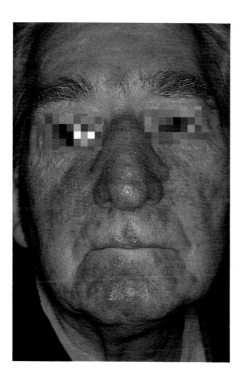

Papulopustular form
Inflamed papules and aseptic pustules appear on a background of telangiectatic erythema, but never comedones (which necessarily leads to rejection of the term "acne rosacea").

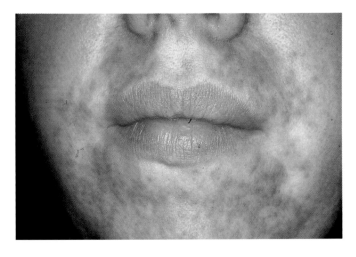

PERIORAL DERMATITIS

This is characterized by the appearance of micropapules and micropustules on a base of erythema and oedema, mainly around the mouth, separated from the lips by a border of healthy skin. The lesions can sometimes spread to the nasolabial folds.

DRUG-INDUCED ERUPTIONS

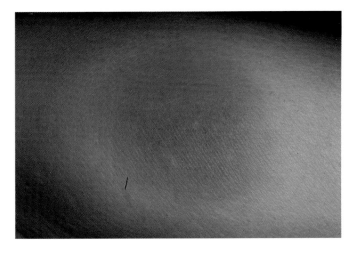

FIXED PIGMENTED ERYTHEMA

Well-circumscribed pigmented erythematous patch occurring 48 h after the ingestion of a drug, in this case phenacetin. The lesion resolves into a residual pigmentation which disappears gradually. Reintroduction of the drug causes a recurrence, invariably at the same site. In some cases the centre of the lesion can be bullous (fixed bullous toxic dermatitis).

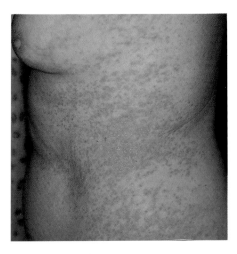

MACULOPAPULAR EXANTHEMA (MORBILLIFORM ERUPTION)

Eruption characterized by dull red congestive patches on the skin. These vary in size and run together into sheets.

Two prominent characteristics are the usual symmetry of the lesions and their itchiness. The present case is an ampicillin rash.

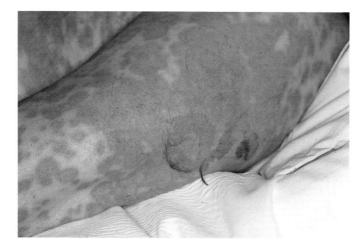

LYELL'S SYNDROME (TOXIC EPIDERMAL NECROLYSIS)

Detachment of large pieces of epidermis, leaving extensive areas of erosion. The eruption usually spreads all over the skin. All mucous membranes are involved in the necrolytic process. The situation is similar to that of major burns.

The drug responsible in this particular case was sulfonamide.

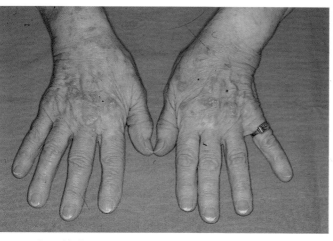

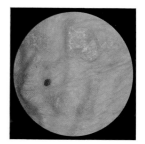

LICHENOID ERUPTIONS

Drug-induced lichenoid eruption caused by methyldopa.
The clinical picture is quite similar to that of lichen planus, but the lesions are often more red and scaly. The distribution of the lesions is symmetrical and more diffuse than in most forms of lichen planus.

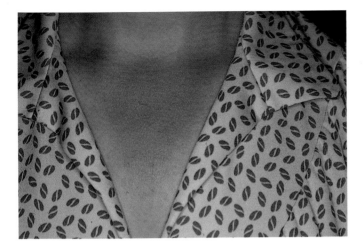

DRUG-INDUCED PHOTOTOXIC ERUPTION

Drug-induced phototoxic eruption associated with the ingestion of a tetracycline. Erythematous oedematous lesions whose pattern corresponds strictly to the skin areas exposed to sunlight. The borders of the lesions are as if "cut with a knife".

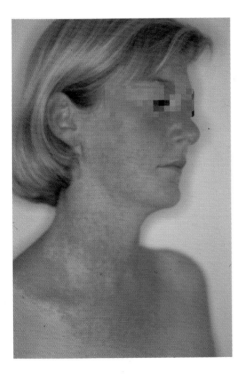

DRUG-INDUCED PHOTOALLERGIC ERUPTION

Drug-induced photoallergic reaction associated with the ingestion of a phenothiazine.
The symptoms comprise erythema, confluent papules, and plaques of weeping vesicular eczema. The lesions, which are accompanied by severe itching, spread beyond the areas exposed to the sun, in contrast to the phototoxic reactions.

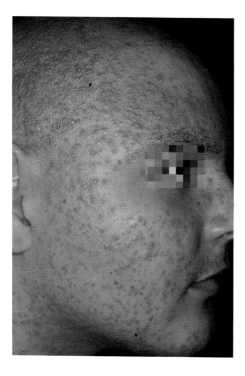

ACNEIFORM FACIAL ERUPTION

This drug-induced eruption is associated in the present case with intramuscular injections of vitamin B12. It is clinically monomorphic, i.e. it is characterized by the presence of papules and pustules and by the absence of comedones.

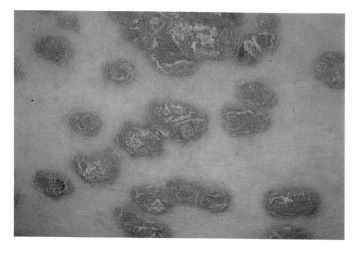

PSORIATIFORM ERUPTION

Psoriatiform eruption associated with the ingestion of a ß-blocker. In certain cases this is an aggravation of existing psoriasis.
The lesions are not usually very scaly. They can be itchy. There is an increasingly large number of suspected groups of drugs.

127

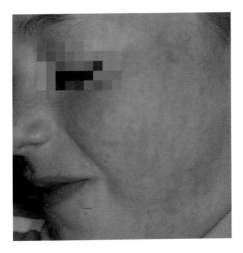

DRUG-INDUCED LUPUS

Induced lupus usually assumes the appearance of subacute or systemic lupus. It is reversible when the treatment is stopped, and recurs if the treatment is reintroduced.

In this case the suspected drug is an anticonvulsant.

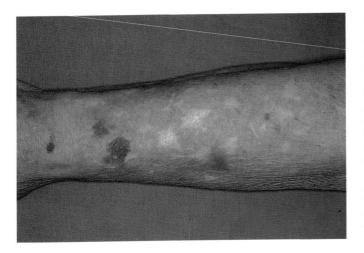

CORTISONE ATROPHY

Prolonged systemic use of corticosteroids leads to a reduction in collagen tissue, culminating in atrophy of the skin. This occurs particularly on the extensor surfaces of the forearms. The atrophy is accompanied by purpura, ecchymoses, and also by these three unusual star-shaped false scars resulting from an internal tear in the dermal tissue (without a wound).

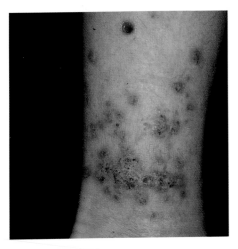

BROMIDE AND IODIDE ERUPTIONS (HALIDE ERUPTIONS)

Very rare reactions to the use of drugs containing bromine or iodine. Bromide and iodide eruptions appear as plaques and lumps with infiltration and vegetation, which are sometimes covered in pustules and crusts. The illustration is of a bromide eruption caused by bromazepam.

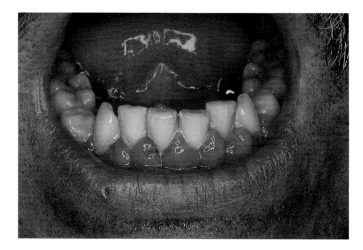

GINGIVAL HYPERPLASIA

Gingival hyperplasias are often provoked by a drug. The drugs most frequently blamed are anticonvulsants (phenytoin, sodium valproate) and cyclosporin, as in the present case.

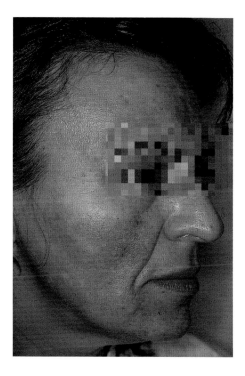

MELASMA (CHLOASMA)

A specifically female skin disease, melasma is hyperpigmentation appearing on the upper part of the face (temples and forehead), but sparing the hairline. It is generally bilateral, but never perfectly symmetrical. Its colour varies from light to dark brown. Melasma occurs in pregnancy or during treatment with hormonal contraceptives. It becomes more pronounced in summer and the aggravating influence of exposure to solar ultraviolet is evident.

SKIN DISORDERS CAUSED BY PHYSICAL AGENTS

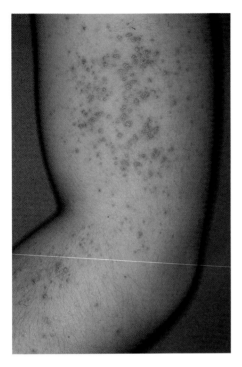

BENIGN SUMMER PHOTODERMATITIS

Small acuminate erythematous papules, a few millimetres in diameter, and papulovesicles clustered on the extensor surface of the arms (as in the present case), legs, and exposed areas of the neck and the chest. The eruption usually spares the face. It occurs a few hours after sunbathing.

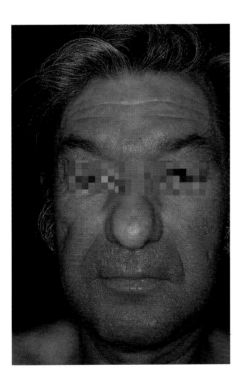

POLYMORPHIC LIGHT ERUPTION

Small erythematous papules or oedematous plaques appearing on exposed parts of the body, especially the face (forehead, nose, cheekbones), behind the ears, the exposed area of neck and chest, and the extensor surfaces of the limbs. In more than 70% of the cases the eruption appears in spring. The patient does not have to be unaccustomed to the sun. The condition appears in the course of everyday life, whether the sky is clear or cloudy.

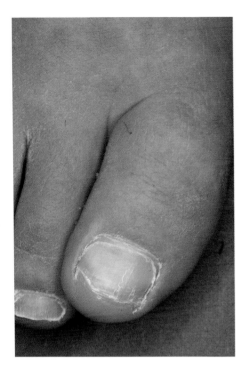

CHILBLAINS

Erythematous and cyanotic infiltrations of the toes which may become covered with clear or haemorrhagic bullae, ulcerations, or small crusts. Chilblains are purple and painful in the cold, but become red and itchy when the sufferer enters a heated room. Chilblains are most common in young women, but they are seen at all ages in both sexes.

Other sites include the heels, ankles, knees, ears, etc.

TOPOGRAPHICAL DERMATOLOGY

ALOPECIA

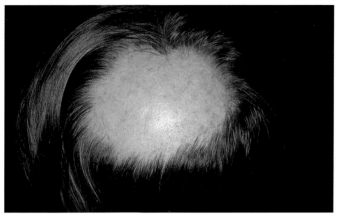

photo 1

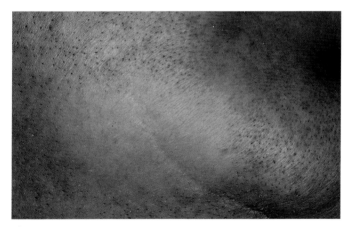

photo 2

ALOPECIA AREATA

Alopecia areata of the scalp is characterized by the appearance of round or oval, smooth, shiny patches of alopecia which gradually increase in size. The patches are usually homogeneously glabrous and are bordered by a peripheral scatter of short broken-off hairs known as exclamation-mark hairs (photo 1). Alopecia areata of the occipital region, known as ophiasis, is more resistant to regrowth. Other hair regions can also be affected: eyebrows, eyelashes, beard (photo 2), and the axillary and pubic regions. In some cases the alopecia can be generalized: this is known as alopecia totalis (scalp) and alopecia universalis (whole body).

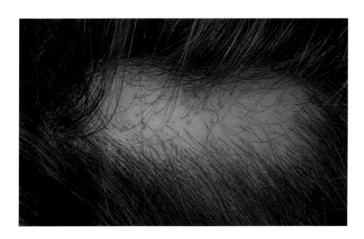

PSEUDOPELADE

Pseudopelade consists of circumscribed alopecia which varies in shape and in size, with more or less distinct limits. The skin is atrophic and adheres to the underlying tissue layers. This unusual cicatricial clinical appearance can be symptomatic of various other conditions: lupus erythematosus, lichen planus, folliculitis decalvans. Some cases are idiopathic and these are known as pseudopelade.

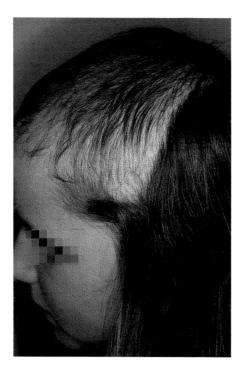

TRICHOTILLOMANIA

Plucking of the hair on a large scale. In trichotillomania the alopecia has irregular, "geographic" margins which may be distinct or indefinite. The area of alopecia can be entirely glabrous or dotted with clumps of broken hairs of very different lengths, and either smooth or covered irregularly with small excoriations or crusts caused by scratching. Similar lesions can appear on the nails (onychotillomania).

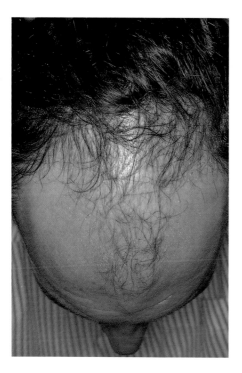

ANDROGENETIC ALOPECIA

This alopecia, known generally as baldness, occurs in adulthood both in men, where it affects the temporal regions (photo) and/or the crown, and in women, where it is confined to the central area of the scalp, in a longitudinal band which extends from the forehead to the crown. In females alopecia always leaves a large number of healthy hairs which are scattered irregularly over the alopecic area.

MUCOSAL DISEASES

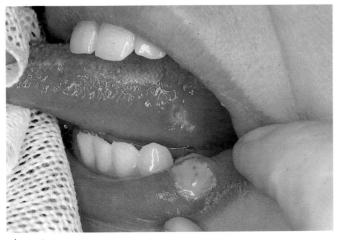

photo 1

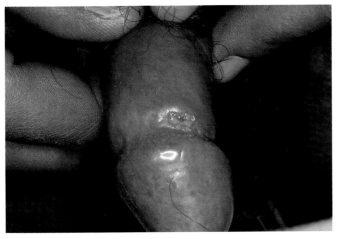

photo 2

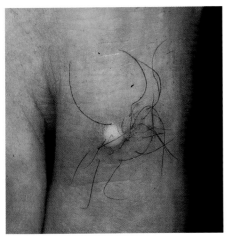

photo 3

APHTHAE, APHTHOSIS, BEHÇET'S DISEASE

Small "punched-out" ulcerations of the buccal mucosa, characterized by a yellowish base resembling the colour of fresh butter and by an erythematous inflammatory halo (photo 1). Often very painful, aphthae are accompanied by lymphadenopathy. Aphthae can occur on the genital mucosa (bipolar aphthosis; photo 2). Behçet's disease is a severe condition with the additional characteristics of aphthae on the skin (photo 3) and an isomorphic reaction to injections.

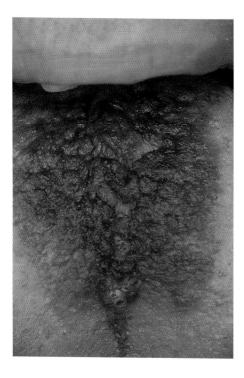

BLACK HAIRY TONGUE

Black hairy tongue comprises hypertrophy of the villi on the upper surface of the tongue. These are loaded with oxidized keratin, which explains the brown or black colour of the lesion. It can occur after the use of certain drugs, such as antibiotics or metronidazole, for example.

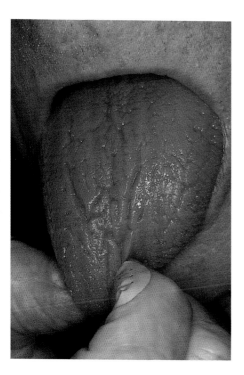

SCROTAL/FISSURED TONGUE

The upper surface of the tongue is criss-crossed by deep grooves running in various directions.
The lingual papillae are often hypertrophic and inflamed. On discovery of this anatomical peculiarity the subjects often complain of a painful sensation (glossodynia).

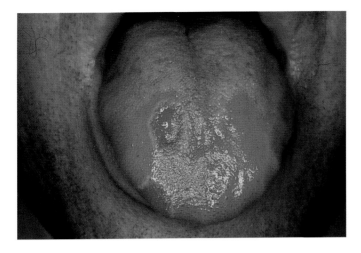

GEOGRAPHIC TONGUE (BENIGN MIGRATORY GLOSSITIS)

Well-defined patches denuded of papillae, surrounded by an unobtrusive whitish border. The spread of these areas is eccentric and their appearance changes from one day to the next.
This could be a variant of lingual psoriasis. Association with scrotal tongue is common.

CHEILITIS

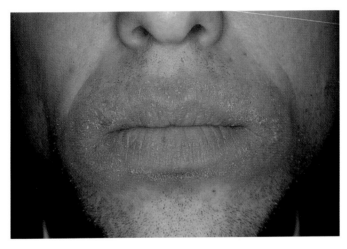

ALLERGIC CONTACT CHEILITIS

Allergic contact dermatitis connected with the application of a lipstick containing balsam of Peru. The eczematous condition extends far beyond the limits of the vermilion zone of the lips, to spread out over the surrounding skin.

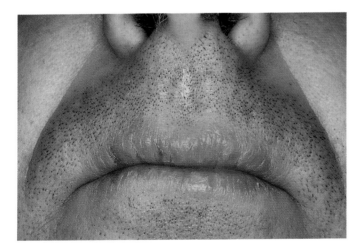

CHEILITIS CAUSED BY SYSTEMIC USE OF ISOTRETINOIN

Cheilitis caused by ingestion of isotretinoin. This is a fissured, scaly, erythematous cheilitis which is dependent on the isotretinoin dose administered. There are sometimes associated episodes of epistaxis.

MISCELLANEOUS

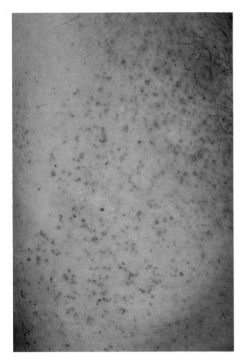

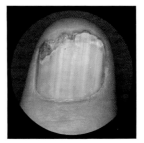

DARIER'S DISEASE
Hereditary skin disease with a characteristic topography (sides of the face, trunk). Multiple small greyish-brown papules are observed, keratotic, dry, and very adherent. These papules can run together to form extensive brownish plaques. The lesions have a very distinct tendency to increase during the months of sunshine.

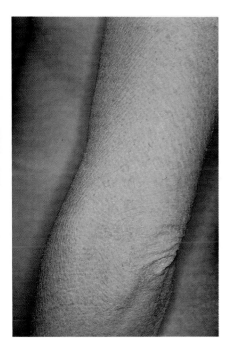

ICHTHYOSIS VULGARIS
Condition transmitted by a dominant gene, sometimes associated with atopic dermatitis. The whole of the skin is affected, sprinkled with small dry scales, which vary in number. Improvement during the months of sunshine is typical. Acquired ichthyosis must always make one think of a paraneoplastic syndrome (e.g. underlying Hodgkin's disease).

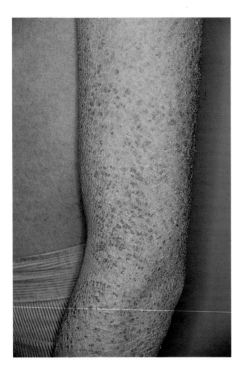

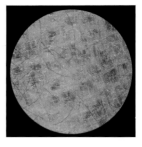

SEX-LINKED (RECESSIVE) ICHTHYOSIS

Also called *ichthyosis nigricans*, this variant of ichthyosis is found only in boys, does not spare the major skin folds, and presents in the form of wide, adherent, blackish scales.

HEREDITARY PALMOPLANTAR KERATODERMA (THOST-UNNA SYNDROME)

Appearing very early in life (between the 4th and 8th week), this palmoplantar keratoderma represents the model of a disease with autosomal dominant transmission. There are extensive yellowish keratotic plaques, accompanied by large cracks in flexural creases of the palms. This keratoderma is distinctly demarcated and does not extend to the wrist. The keratotic lesions are accentuated by an inflammatory border. There is sometimes associated hyperhidrosis.

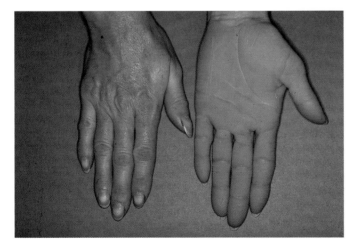

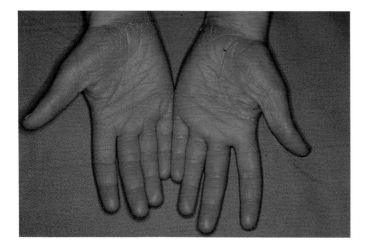

PITYRIASIS RUBRA PILARIS

Association of diffuse orange-yellow palmoplantar keratoderma with a scoring of small fissures and horny follicular papules producing a grid on the skin. On palpation it feels abrasive (like emery paper). The pinkish papules are pointed at the top and surmounted by a small horny follicular plug.

The course is usually chronic. Episodes of erythroderma may be seen as time goes on.

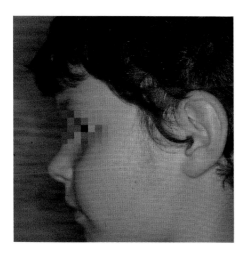

KERATOSIS PILARIS

Extremely common skin disease surrounded by a fine erythematous border, characterized by slight hyperkeratosis of the hair follicle orifices.

This "condition" is transmitted by an autosomal dominant gene and is usually seen on the cheeks and the temples. In adults the exterior surfaces of the arms and anterior surfaces of the thigh are most frequently affected. The affected areas feel abrasive on palpation. Exposure to sunlight attenuates the condition.

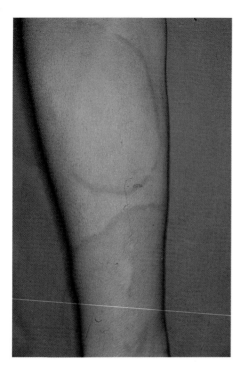

ERYTHEMA ANNULARE CENTRIFUGUM (DARIER'S)

Extensive annular lesions of the arms with the appearance of healing at the centre. The distinctly infiltrated erythematous margins spread slowly outwards. Having appeared suddenly, this condition has become chronic, each ring developing over several weeks at a rate of 2 to 3 mm per week. It should be noted that when two rings join together they never overlap. There is no pruritus. It is always important to check for a possible underlying cause, though in a number of cases erythema annulare centrifugum remains idiopathic. Among the potential causes the following should be remembered: remote infectious foci, viral diseases, Hodgkin's disease, visceral cancer, autoimmune thyroiditis, lupus erythematosus, liver disease, etc.
In the present case it was viral hepatitis B which, after an acute episode, subsequently developed into chronic active hepatitis.

LEG ULCERS

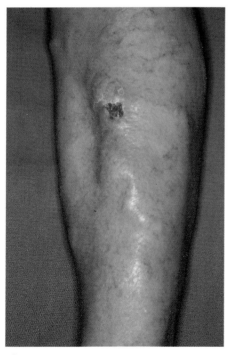

VENOUS LEG ULCER

Extensive ulceration with pliant borders and outlines which vary from one case to the next. The base of the ulcer is granular in some places and sanious and necrotic in others. Surrounding trophic disorders are evident: gravitational purpura, atrophie blanche. This type of ulcer can be the result of a varicose disorder or a postphlebitic syndrome. It represents more than 80% of leg ulcer cases. It affects women most frequently and there is an evident hereditary factor. The pains vary individually in intensity and are improved by lying down.

photo 1

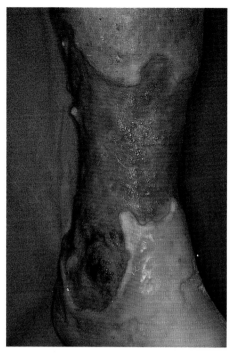

photo 2

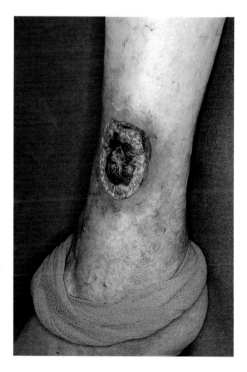

ISCHAEMIC (ARTERIAL) LEG ULCER

Punched-out ulceration which is most often unilateral. Its site is near the ankle. There is no associated trophic disorder. The pulse in the foot can be felt only with difficulty. Ischaemic ulcers develop rapidly and cause intense pain which is often aggravated by lying down. They are much less common than venous ulcers and can be found in diabetes, arteriosclerosis, or Buerger's disease.

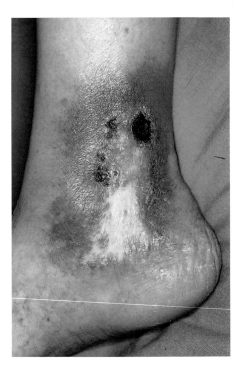

ULCER CAUSED BY CAPILLARITIS

Slow and relatively superficial ulceration with jagged and irregular margins. There is surrounding pigmentary and purpuric angiodermatitis, sometimes associated with small patches of atrophie blanche. The pains are often intense and persistent, and are not influenced by lying down. Diabetes and arteriosclerosis promote this condition.

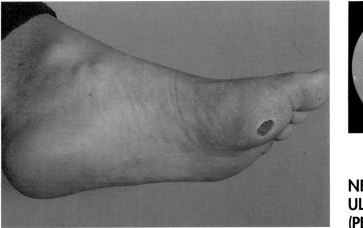

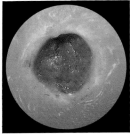

NEUROTROPHIC LEG ULCER (PERFORATING ULCER)

Deep circular, punched-out ulcer found at the bearing surface of the metatarsal joint. The base is necrotic. There is no tendency towards spontaneous cicatrization. There is virtually no pain. In the present case it is caused by diabetes with a major neuropathological component. Other neurological conditions can be responsible (e.g. syringomyelia).

PATHOMIMICRY

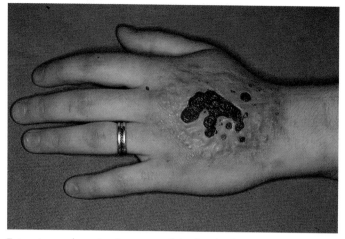

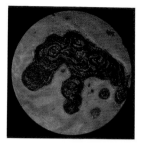

SKIN SELF-MUTILATION, SIMULATED DISEASE

Extensive escharotic ulceration of the back of the hand, caused intentionally with caustic soda. The margins are distinct, the angular edges and the configuration "surprising". The appearance of the lesion was very rapid and recurrences at the same site are typical. The course is usually capricious, spontaneous healing retarded, and persistence indefinite. In the present case the patient acted voluntarily with intent to deceive, for her own advantage (extension of sick leave from work).

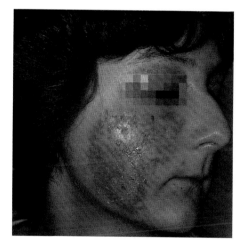

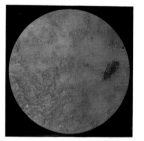

SELF-MUTILATION, PATHOMIMICRY

Ulceration of exogenous origin on the face, with distinct margins and "aberrant" configuration. This particular topography is rarely found in cases of disease simulation. True pathomimicry is caused by the patient who is "unconscious" of it or shows "dual consciousness". Major psychological disturbances are present. There is no evident intention to take financial advantage of the condition.

SKIN TUMOURS
A. Benign

EPIDERMAL TUMOURS

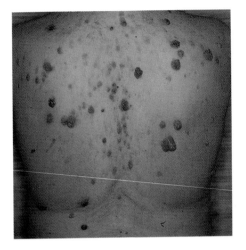

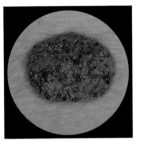

SEBORRHOEIC KERATOSIS/WART
Excrescences of varying size, covered with a greasy, scaly keratotic layer which is not very adherent. They can have various colours: yellow, sepia, grey, dark brown, or pure black.
Each lesion seems to be "placed" on the skin surface, is well-circumscribed, has no underlying infiltration.

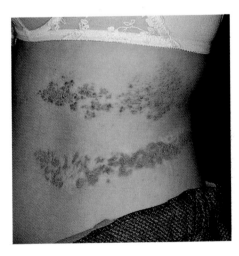

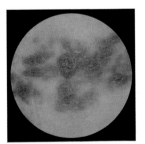

VERRUCOUS EPIDERMAL NAEVUS
The epidermal naevus appears in the form of raised papuloverrucous lesions, rough to the touch and sometimes fragmented. It is usually disposed in continuous linear bands following the Blaschko's classical lines, to be interrupted over the midline.
The colour is that of normal skin, sometimes greyish or brownish.

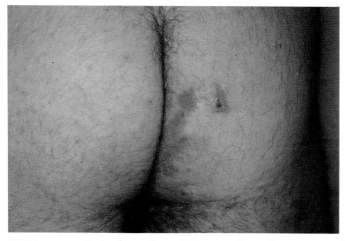
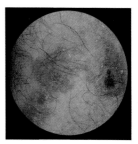

INFLAMMATORY LINEAR VERRUCOUS EPIDERMAL NAEVUS (ILVEN)

ILVEN appears in the form of psoriatiform scaly erythematous patches, which are sometimes lichenoid or verrucous, disposed in linear bands following Blaschko's lines (like the lesions of verrucous epidermal naevus).

Inflammatory episodes can occur, causing exacerbation of pruritus, more or less severe excoriations, secondary eczematization, and even areas of necrosis.

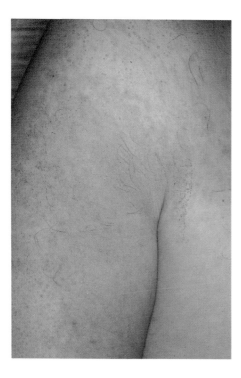

BECKER'S NAEVUS (PIGMENTED AND HAIRY EPIDERMAL NAEVUS)

Hyperpigmented unilateral plaque, the preferred site of which is the chest or the shoulder, sometimes covered in hairs. It appears most often in young adults after exposure to the sun.

It corresponds to a late epithelial (epidermal and follicular) naevus with secondary epidermal melanin hyperpigmentation.

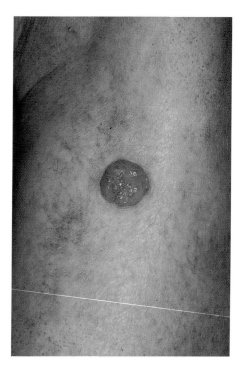

CLEAR CELL ACANTHOMA
Small, round and domed firm tumour, which is generally isolated, pink in colour, usually with a moist surface.
The diagnosis of this lesion is essentially histopathological.

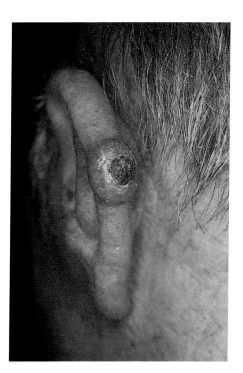

KERATO-ACANTHOMA
Very well defined nodule surmounted by a central horny plug. Its growth is rapid, the maximum size of the lesion being reached in a few weeks.
The lesion usually regresses spontaneously in a few months.

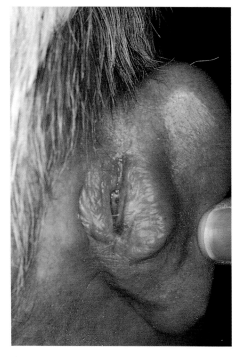

photo 1

SPECTACLE FRAME ACANTHOMA (FISSURED ACANTHOMA)

Well-circumscribed, slightly pink retro-auricular papulonodule, 1-2 cm in diameter, surrounded by an inflammatory halo (photo 1). The lesion is divided in two by a groove (fold).

Acanthoma occurs in the weeks or months after the patient starts wearing a new spectacle frame (photo 2).

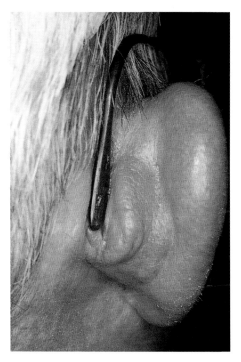

photo 2

FOLLICULAR AND SEBACEOUS TUMOURS

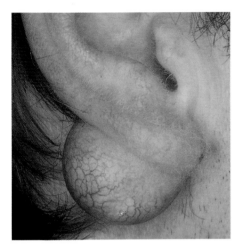

EPIDERMOID CYST

Inflammatory subcutaneous nodule, often with a punctiform opening at its centre, through which malodorous whitish or yellowish material can be expressed.

It is a single or multiple lesion which occurs especially in seborrhoeic areas, within the context of acne vulgaris or nodulocystic acne. Epidermoid cysts are sometimes wrongly called "sebaceous cysts".

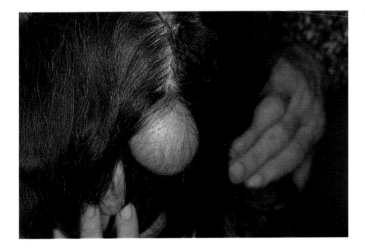

TRICHILEMMAL CYST (PILAR CYST)

Generally located on the scalp, it appears in the form of a subcutaneous nodule covered with non-adherent pink and glabrous skin. The cysts are sometimes multiple. They range from pea-size to egg-size and are colloquially known as wens.

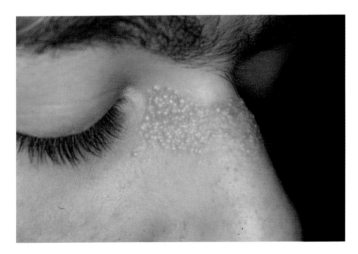

MILIA

Milia are very superficial small white elevations which occur in various circumstances. In newborn babies they appear as innumerable small white dots on the face, as illustrated in the photograph, caused by transient retention of sebum. They disappear spontaneously in a few weeks. In adolescents and adults they are commonly seen on the cheeks, the eyelids, and the nose, and are due to clogging of follicles.

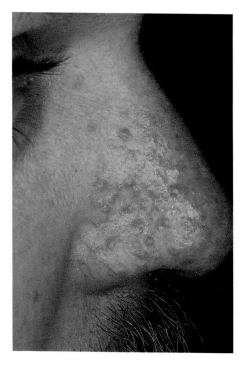

TRICHOEPITHELIOMA

Translucent, flattened or globular papular formations, 2 to 5 mm in diameter, pink or white in colour and sometimes surmounted by fine telangiectasias. Their preferred site is the face (nose, nasolabial folds, cheeks, forehead, chin). These are generally multiple and hereditary lesions, appearing from childhood or in adolescence.

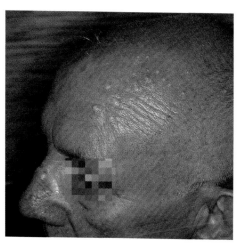

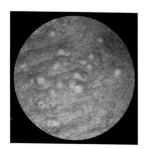

SENILE SEBACEOUS ADENOMA

Small yellowish umbilicate formations, 3 to 6 mm in diameter, occurring on seborrhoeic areas of the face (forehead, temples, cheeks) in both sexes after the age of fifty. These adenomas correspond to senile adenomatous hyperplasia of the sebaceous glands.

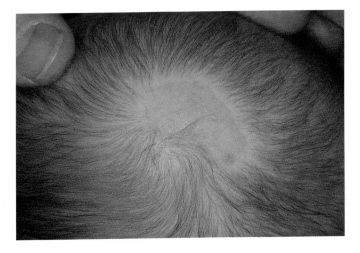

JADASSOHN'S SEBACEOUS NAEVUS

This is a tumour on the scalp or the face, which is often congenital. Its appearance changes with age. During childhood there is an oval or pink and slightly raised alopecic plaque. Starting from puberty the surface becomes mamillated and warty, and assumes the characteristic orange-yellow colour. In adulthood it can, in exceptional cases, give rise to a basal-cell carcinoma.

SWEAT GLAND TUMOURS

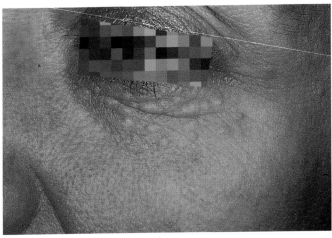

SYRINGOMA

Small, always multiple lesions measuring 1 to 3 mm in diameter and forming smooth, flesh-coloured papules generally occurring on the face (especially the eyelids), chest, neck, and axillae.

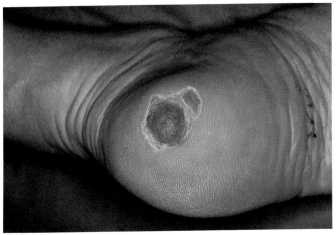

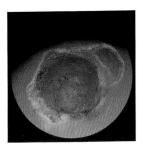

ECCRINE POROMA

Solitary benign congestive tumour bleeding in pinpoint haemorrhages, the wide base of which is encircled by a keratin collar. Its preferred site is the area of the sole around the heel. In differential diagnostics it must be distinguished from pyogenic granuloma and achromic malignant melanoma.

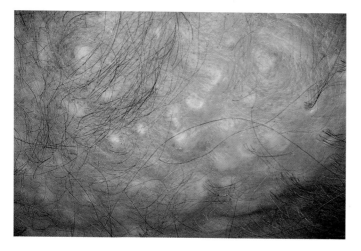

CYLINDROMA

Multiple benign tumours, often familial, appearing on the scalp, which becomes mamillated and embossed (turban-like tumours).
The surface of these tumours is smooth, glabrous, normal or pink in colour, with telangiectasias. There is no adherence to deep layers.

CONNECTIVE TISSUE TUMOURS

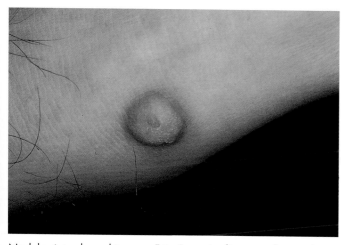

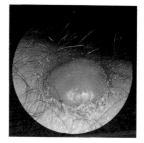

DERMATOFIBROMA

Nodular intradermal tumour 5 to 6 mm in diameter, firm to the touch, generally located on the legs. Its surface is pigmented to varying degree and often slightly keratotic. A dermatofibroma can sometimes be caused by an insect bite. An unusual variant is the pastille-like fibroma, a pink shiny nodule with a smooth surface surrounded by a very fine scaly collarette separated from the tumour by a groove.

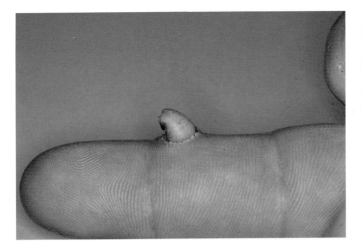

ACQUIRED DIGITAL FIBROKERATOMA

Small tumour situated on the fingers or toes, more rarely on the palms and soles. Like the pastille fibroma, it is a solitary domed lesion, sometimes elongated and pedunculate, surrounded by a fine demarcating border. The surface is slightly warty. It is perhaps caused by a trauma.

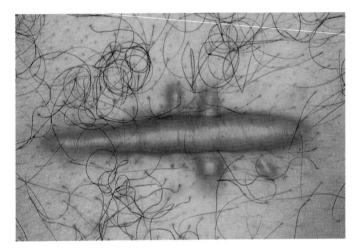

KELOID

Red and taut fibrous tumour with a smooth surface, slightly dented and sometimes surrounded by pseudopodia-like extensions called crab legs. They are very often itchy, painful, or tender.

Post-traumatic keloids secondary to **wounds, burns, vaccinations**, or inflammatory skin lesions (such as **adolescent acne**) are distinguished from **spontaneous keloids**, which are more common in black people.

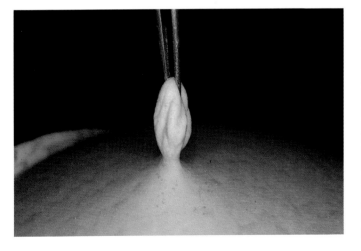

SKIN TAG (ACROCHORDON, MOLLUSCUM PENDULUM)

Small and very soft fleshy mass, on average 3 to 5 mm in diameter, implanted in the skin by a thin stalk. These lesions are often multiple and their preferred sites are the axillae or inguinal flexures, the neck, the eyelids, and the orbital area.

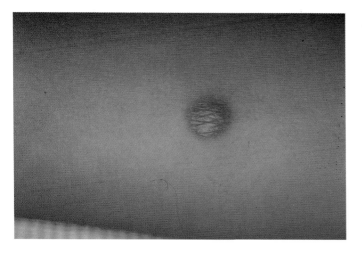

JUVENILE XANTHOGRANULOMA

Single or multiple papulonodular yellow, orange or brown lesion of soft consistency, usually appearing on the face, scalp, trunk, and the base of the limbs. It occurs most frequently in neonates and infants, but can also be seen in children and even in adults.

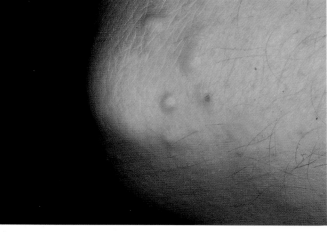

photo 1

TUBEROUS XANTHOMA

Small hemispherical papules, from a few millimetres to a centimetre in diameter, pink or orange in colour, sometimes very yellow (photo 1) on vitropression. The preferred sites are the elbows, knees, and buttocks. A rare variant (eruptive xanthoma) (photo 2) is found in cases of severe hyper-triglyceridaemia.

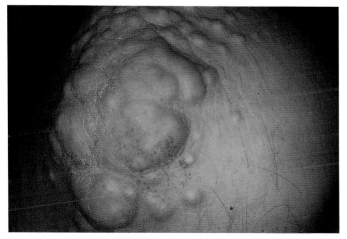

photo 2

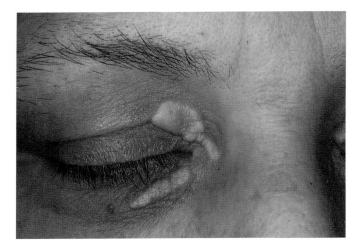

XANTHELASMA PALPEBRARUM
Flattened and clearly delimited yellowish or orange plaques around the eyes. This is one of the variants of xanthoma planum.

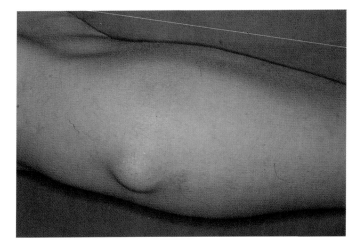

LIPOMA
Single or multiple benign tumours the colour of normal skin, which develop from subcutaneous fat. They are soft in consistency and they can attain a large size.

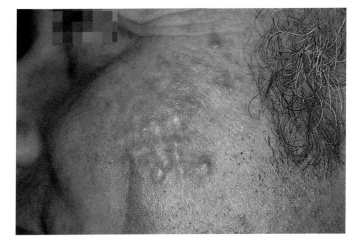

LEIOMYOMA
Benign tumours originating from the smooth muscles connected with hair follicles, genitals, nipples, or blood vessels. Leiomyomas are single or multiple, contractile, nodular tumours, which are red, pink, or brownish in colour.

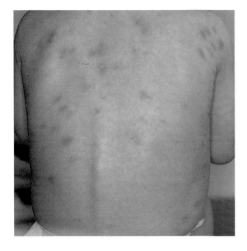

CUTANEOUS MASTOCYTOSIS

The term mastocytosis covers all lesions caused by the proliferation of mast cells in skin.

Urticaria pigmentosa

This is the most common form, encountered in all age groups. It produces a fairly monomorphic eruption of smooth violet or brown itchy macules or maculopapules. The reactivity of the lesions to certain stimuli, such as rubbing, is very characteristic (Darier's sign).

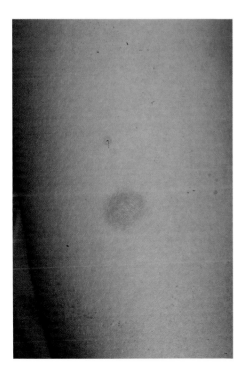

Mastocytoma

Single firm tumour, orange in colour, occurring only in children.

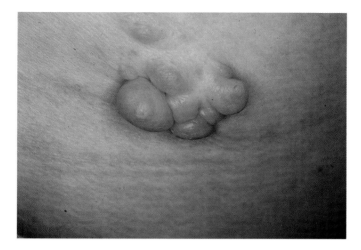

NEURAL CREST DISEASES

Neurofibroma

Nodules which are of normal skin colour or pink. Their firmness can vary. Their essential characteristic is that they are readily depressible.

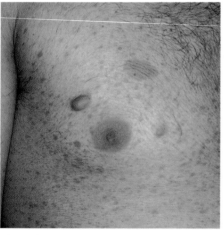

photo 1

Neurofibromatosis 1 (von Recklinghausen neurofibromatosis)

This is the most common form of systemic neural crest disease. It is essentially characterized by the combination of café au lait spots, "freckling", and cutaneous neurofibromas (photo 1). The "principal tumour" is a neurofibroma which is very large (photo 2) in relation to all those surrounding it.

This hereditary condition is transmitted by an autosomal dominant gene with high penetrance and variable expression.

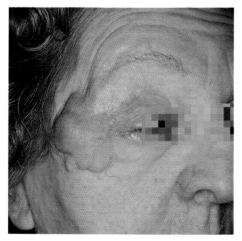

photo 2

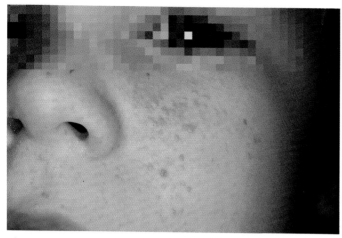

photo 1

Bourneville's tuberous sclerosis (epiloia)

Tuberous sclerosis is a condition with autosomal dominant transmission, characterized by various isolated or associated clinical signs and symptoms.

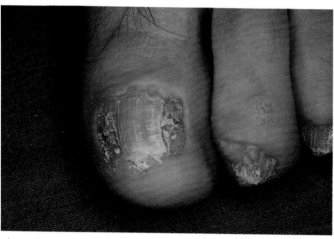

photo 2

a. **Angiofibroma**
   Small, firm, pink or red tumid nodules covered in fine telangiectases and distributed symmetrically over the face: nasolabial folds, cheeks, perioral region (photo 1).
b. **Periungual fibromas (Koënen's tumours)**
   Very rare horny angiofibromas of the toes (photo 2).

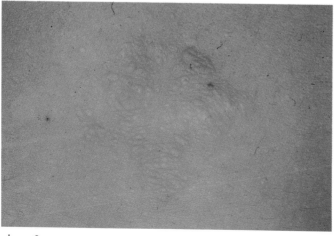

photo 3

c. **Shagreen patch**
   Raised patch with an irregular outline and surface, covered with pale "orange-skin". Its preferred site is the lumbosacral region (photo 3).
d. **Achromic patches**
   Fairly regular macules 1 to 10 cm in diameter, oval, rounded, or more characteristically in the shape of an ash leaf. They are white and do not have a hyperaemic or pigmented halo.

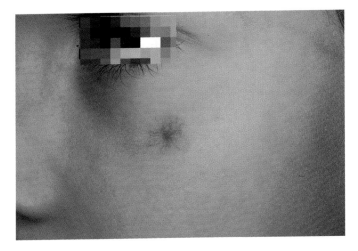

ANGIOMA
Spider telangiectasis
Vascular star, composed of a red central point, sometimes raised and pulsatile, and arborizations radiating outwards.
The arborizations disappear on vitropression.

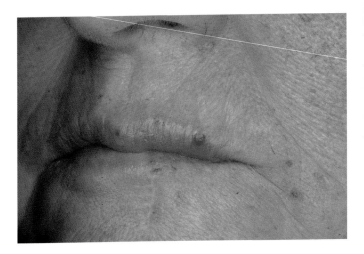

Hereditary haemorrhagic telangiectasia (Osler-Rendu-Weber disease)
Autosomal dominant disease, characterized by telangiectases of the skin and mucous membranes, often not appearing until after puberty.
The telangiectatic macules are poorly defined and the arborizations, in contrast to spider telangiectasis, are not symmetrical. They occur predominantly on the face, hands, buccal mucosa, the lips, and the tongue.

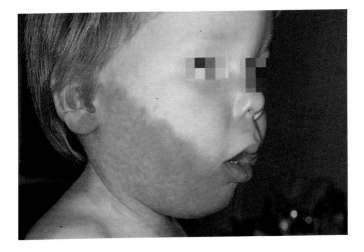

Angioma planum
Congenital erythematous macule of varying intensity, extent, and shape.
The colour varies from pale pink to dark red. Its preferred site is the face and the limbs, but it can spread to the mucosa. From the fourth decade of life the angioma thickens and superficial violet nodules can appear.

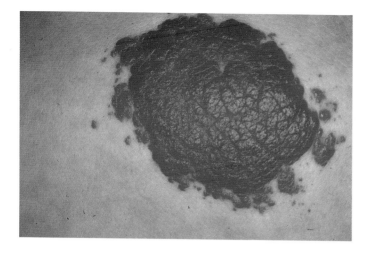

Tuberous angioma

Bright red, distinctly demarcated, raised angioma in infants, projecting above the surrounding normal skin. Its growth is rapid, and it can bleed and ulcerate. Most of these angiomas disappear spontaneously in childhood, leaving no trace.

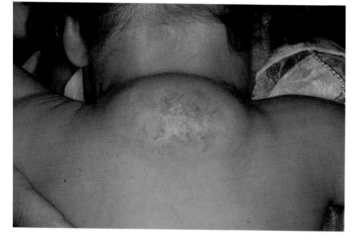

Subcutaneous angioma

Tumour protruding under skin which is either normal, bluish, or telangiectatic. This lesion does not undergo spontaneous involution.

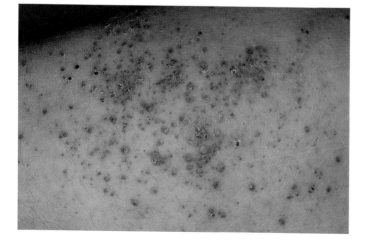

Angiokeratoma

Papular telangiectasia with a hyperkeratotic surface. Angiokeratomas of the scrotum and vulva are the most common. They are usually benign. Nevertheless, if they have disseminated over the buttocks, one must investigate for Fabry's disease.

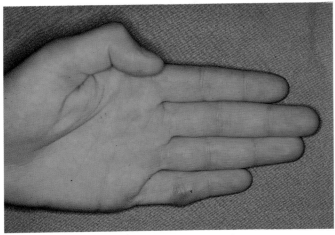
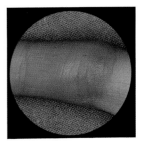

Glomus tumour

Small, bluish intradermal tumour, remarkable for its painfulness. Its site is most likely to be peripheral, on the hands and feet, more rarely on the forearms and buttocks. A common and characteristic site is the subungual region.

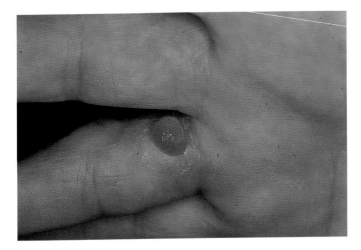

Pyogenic granuloma
Fleshy vascular pimple secondary to minimal or unnoticed trauma. Its eroded surface bleeds easily. Pyogenic granuloma may be "nipped" at its base by a characteristic groove which separates it from neighbouring skin.

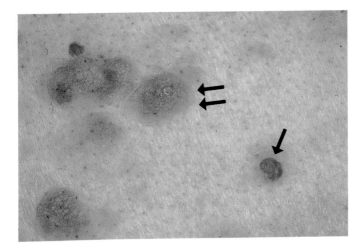

Senile angioma (cherry angioma)
Small bright red patches, flat or slightly tumid. Extremely common in old people, usually multiple and found on the trunk (→). In many cases they coexist with seborrhoeic warts (keratoses) (⇉).

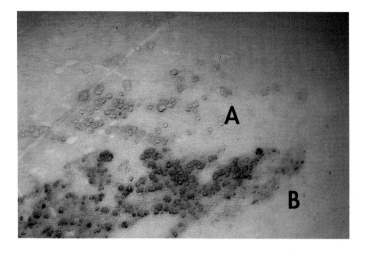

LYMPHANGIOMA

Pseudovesicular elevations 1 to 5 mm in diameter, arranged in clusters or irregular plaques, translucent and taut but readily depressible. The lesions can occur anywhere on the body, but are more commonly found on the trunk and the base of the limbs. Lymphangioma (A) is very often found concomitantly with hemangionma (B) (see photograph).

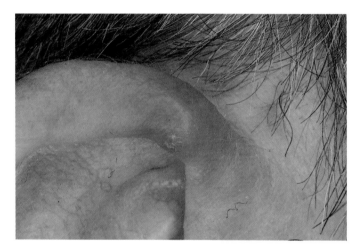

CHONDRODERMATITIS NODULARIS HELICIS

(painful nodule in the ear) Inflammatory nodule of the helix, which is painful or tender. Its centre is keratotic or crater-like. It is nowadays regarded as a chondrodermatitis, but its aetiology has not been clarified.

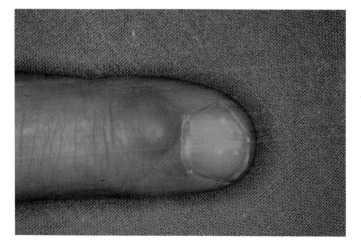

MUCOID PSEUDOCYST

Small, firm, flesh-coloured translucent nodule, occurring on the backs of the fingers near the distal interphalangeal joints and often causing a characteristic nail deformation with longitudinal grooves. It is the result of the accumulation of a mucoid substance in the dermis.

MELANOCYTIC NAEVI

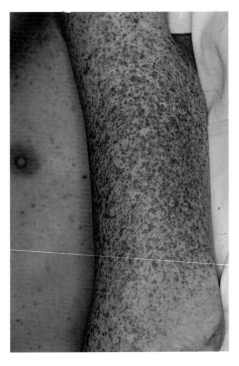

LENTIGO
Small (1 to 3 mm) brown or black hyperpigmented macules which can be distributed all over the skin and/or mucous membranes. Lentigines are often isolated. Sometimes they are generalized (lentiginosis) and form part of complex syndromes involving several internal organs. They represent epidermal hypermelanocytosis.

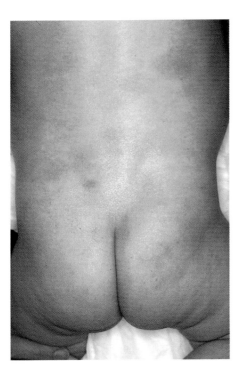

MONGOLIAN SPOT
Bluish grey macules varying in size from a few millimetres to tens of centimetres and occurring most frequently on the loins and buttocks. They are especially common in Orientals. These spots represent dermal hypermelanocytosis.

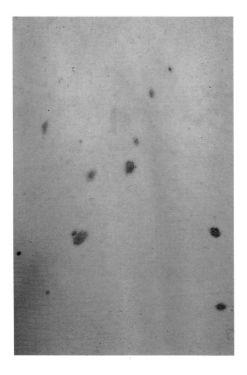

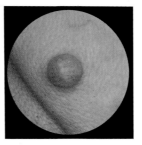

MELANOCYTIC NAEVI (NAEVOCYTIC NAEVI)

Melanocytic naevi are well-circumscribed lesions which show a wide variety of colour, shape, thickness, consistency, and size, their diameter ranging from a few millimetres to a few centimetres. They can be flat or raised, lenticular or discoid, and vary in colour from pale yellow to black-brown. The domed forms may be without pigmentation.

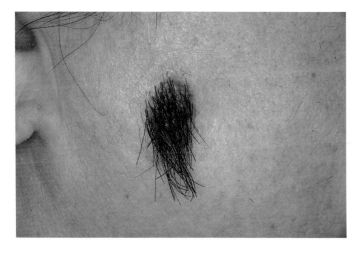

HAIRY MELANOCYTIC NAEVUS

Some melanocytic naevi become covered in hairs at puberty.

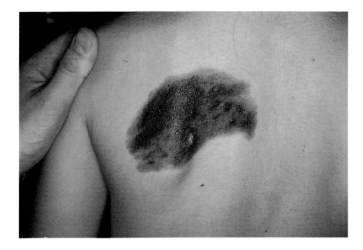

CONGENITAL PIGMENTED NAEVUS

Congenital pigmented naevi vary in size. Some are called giant because of their wide spread. They have an inhomogeneous surface (flat, papular, nodular, verrucous) and are most often variegated in colour, which ranges from light brown to black. They are often covered with thick hairs.

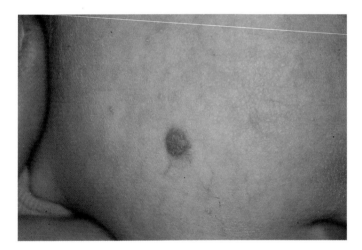

SPITZ NAEVUS (JUVENILE)

Isolated pinkish papulonodular tumour, frequently located on the face or the limbs.
The histopathological appearance of this melanocytic naevus is very characteristic. In fairly exceptional cases there may be multiple Spitz naevi.

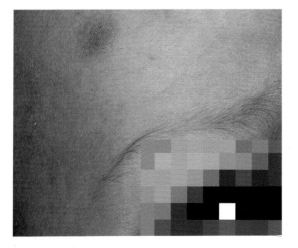

BLUE NAEVUS

Small nodule, often less than a centimetre in diameter, blue-grey to black-blue in colour and situated especially frequently on the back of the hands and the feet, sometimes on the face. Its colour is caused by the deep dermal site of the melanocytic clusters.

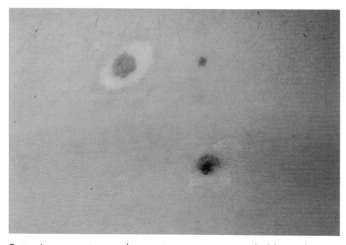
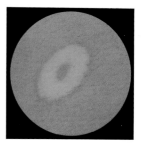

HALO NAEVUS (SUTTON'S NAEVUS)

Sutton's naevus is a melanocytic naevus surrounded by a depigmented corona. In the course of its natural development the naevus component gradually disappears and the white halo undergoes gradual repigmentation. This feature of its course is probably autoimmune.

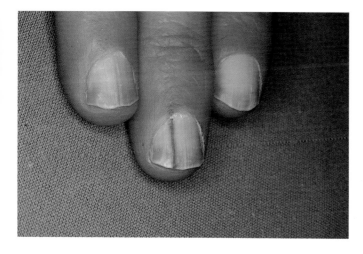

NAEVUS OF THE NAILS

Presence of a more or less dark brown longitudinal band in the nail plate (melanonychia), clinical evidence of the existence of a melanocytic naevus in the matrix region.

B. Premalignant

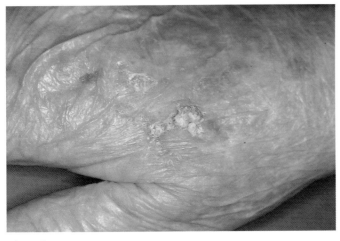

photo 1

SOLAR KERATOSES (SENILE KERATOSES)

Raised red and well-defined plaques with a rough surface covered in scales of varying thickness. The lesions are isolated or multiple and their preferred site is on exposed regions such as the back of the hands (photo 1) or the face (photo 2).

Here one can observe some characteristics of skin-ageing caused by sunlight: sallow skin, accentuated wrinkles, etc.

If left untreated, some cases of solar keratosis develop into squamous cell carcinoma.

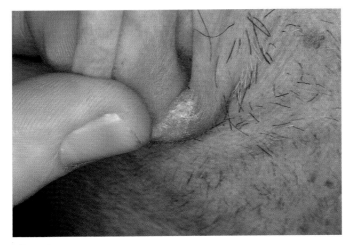

photo 2

ACTINIC CHEILITIS

Relatively well-demarcated scaly erythematous plaque, sometimes encrusted and occurring essentially on the lower lip. Under the hyperkeratotic layer the epithelium is atrophic and bleeds easily at the slightest trauma. Actinic cheilitis spreads slowly over time and can degenerate into true squamous cell carcinoma.

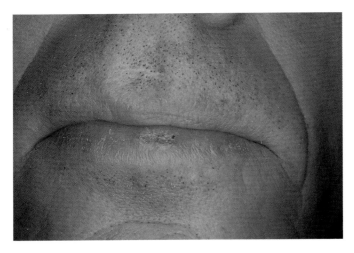

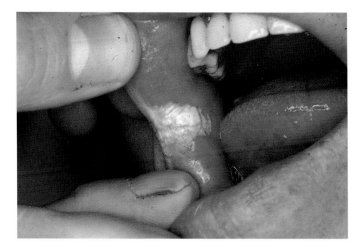

LEUCOPLAKIA - SMOKER'S KERATOSIS (STOMATITIS NICOTINA)

Well-demarcated and more or less rounded white or greyish plaques on the lower lip or the buccal mucosa. They occur more frequently in men and are probably promoted by smoking. Their natural evolution is in the direction of squamous cell carcinoma.

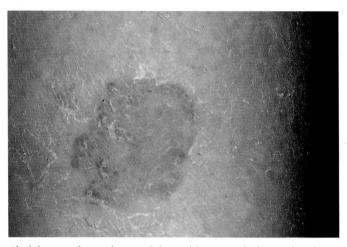

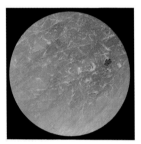

BOWEN'S DISEASE

Slightly raised round or oval discoid lesion with distinct borders, varying in size, red or reddish brown in colour and covered with a crust of scales or with small crusts. The current understanding of Bowen's disease is that it is an intraepidermal carcinoma (*in situ*).

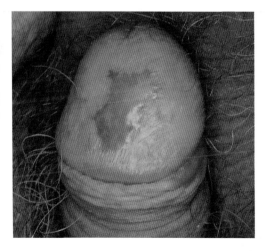

ERYTHROPLASIA OF QUEYRAT

Mucosal site of Bowen's disease. Red, well-demarcated, slightly protuberant plaque, with a glazed surface, on the glans penis. Similar lesions are observed on the vulval mucosa.

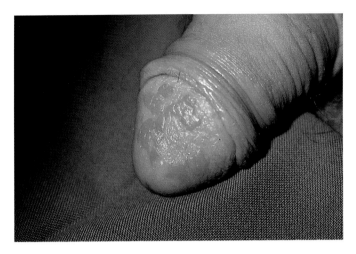

BOWENOID PAPULOSIS

Erythematous or brownish papules on the glans and shaft of the penis, the vulva, and sometimes the perianal region. Their histopathology is similar to that of Bowen's disease. Human papillomaviruses (16,18,33) are the initial cause of this papulosis.

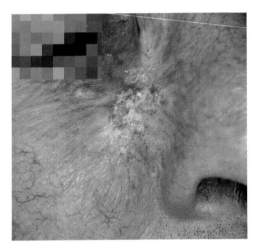

RADIODERMATITIS

Cicatricial atrophy, telangiectases, and pigmentation abnormalities form the classical picture of radiodermatitis. At a further stage ulcerations can appear. Basal cell carcinoma or squamous cell carcinoma are liable to develop after several years.

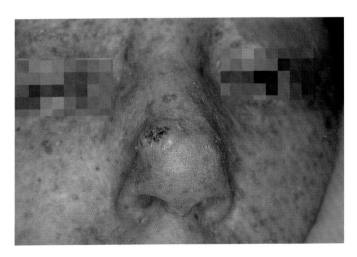

XERODERMA PIGMENTOSUM

A hereditary disease with recessive autosomal transmission. The genetic basis of xeroderma pigmentosum is an enzyme deficiency resulting in disorders of DNA repair after ultraviolet irradiation. The condition is characterized by extreme photosensitivity and chronic actinic lesions including skin atrophy, freckles, and solar keratosis. Some tumours can develop early: kerato-acanthoma, basal cell or squamous cell carcinoma, malignant melanoma.

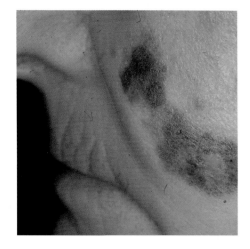

DUBREUILH'S MELANOSIS (LENTIGO MALIGNA MELANOMA, MELANOSIS CIRCUMSCRIPTA PRECANCEROSA OF DUBREUILH)

Polychromatic pigmented macule, not raised and poorly defined.

Its colour varies from pale beige to black. Dubreuilh's melanosis is observed in old people, most frequently on the face, less so on the back of the hands and on the legs. It spreads very slowly, reaching a diameter of several centimetres in about ten years.

C. Malignant

BASAL CELL CARCINOMAS

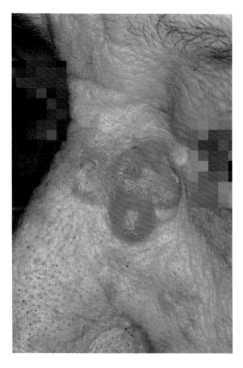

NODULAR BASAL CELL CARCINOMA

Globular tumour with a waxy or reddish tint, more or less translucent ("pearly" carcinoma), the smooth surface of which is streaked with fine telangiectases.

The most common site is the face, but other areas can also be involved: back, limbs, genital region. Nodular basal cell carcinoma increases gradually in size and can ulcerate.

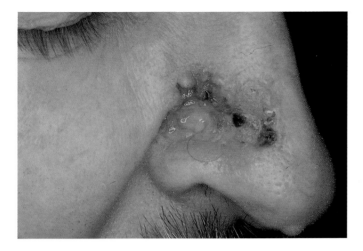

RODENT ULCER

This variant of ulcerated basal cell carcinoma is characterized by

1. an ulcer as the primary lesion
2. considerable superficial spread
3. considerable spread in depth: the tumour "eats" into the tissue (hence "rodent ulcer")
4. the persistence of a translucent pearly and slightly telangiectatic border is very characteristic of basal cell carcinoma.

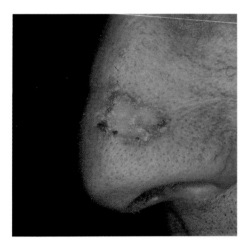

FLAT CICATRICIAL BASAL CELL CARCINOMA ("SCLERODERMA-LIKE" CARCINOMA)

This variant of carcinoma appears more like a plaque than a nodule. The whole central area of the lesion is white, atrophic, sclerous, and morphoea-like, but unlike morphoea it is streaked with telangiectases.

At the edge of the lesion there is usually a pearly, telangiectatic, indurated swelling, sometimes covered with small crusts.

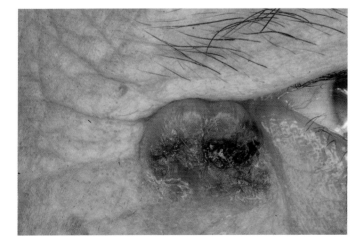

PIGMENTED BASAL CELL CARCINOMA

A very rare variant, pigmented basal cell carcinoma is characterized by a considerable excess of melanin. It is usually nodular and is not ulcerated.

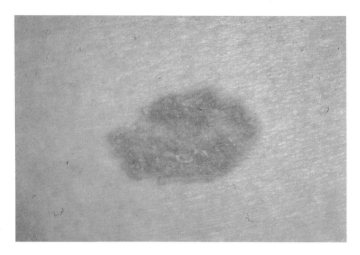

PAGETOID BASAL CELLULAR CARCINOMA (SUPERFICIAL BASAL CELL CARCINOMA)

The usual appearance is a pink plaque distinctly circumscribed by rounded outlines. Its limits are usually marked by a fine, pearly, filiform edge, which distinguishes it from Bowen's disease. Growth is very slow. The preferred site of this variant is on the trunk.

SQUAMOUS CELL CARCINOMAS

The majority of squamous cell carcinomas are seen on uncovered areas: face (lower lip in particular) and the back of the hands. They develop either in apparently healthy skin, or, most frequently, over a precancerous lesion: solar keratosis, Bowen's disease, etc.
They are liable to metastasize, mainly via lymph.

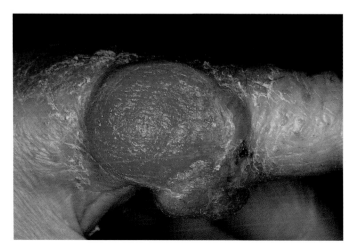

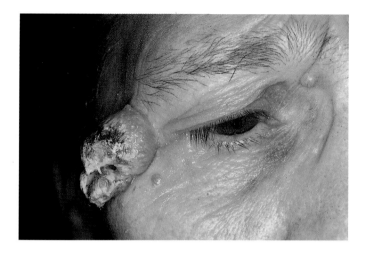

SQUAMOUS CELL CARCINOMA OF THE FACE

Large, ulcerated, which oozes blood and forms crusts. The peripheral swelling is very indurated. The base of the whole lesion is distinctly infiltrated.

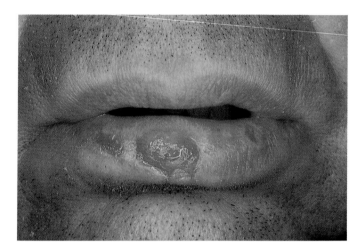

SQUAMOUS CELL CARCINOMA OF THE LOWER LIP

This sanious ulceration is surrounded by an indurated peripheral swelling. In the present case it is developing from actinic cheilitis.

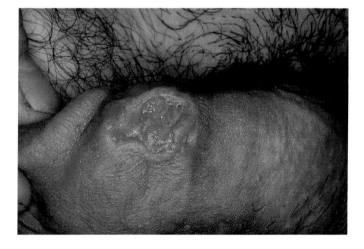

SQUAMOUS CELL CARCINOMA OF THE PENIS

Hard ulcerated vegetating tumour of the glans.

PAGET'S DISEASE

Encrusted scaly erythematous and locally erosive plaque on the nipple and the areola. Its perfectly defined border distinguishes it from an eczematous reaction (see page 24). The disappearance of the nipple's elevation must also be noted. This carcinoma is seen in 3 to 5% of breast cancers and develops mainly in postmenopausal women. Extramammary sites are rare and confined to skin areas with apocrine sweat glands (genitals, perineum, perianal region).

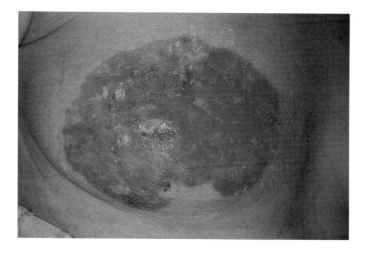

CUTANEOUS METASTASES

Cutaneous metastases of deep cancers can assume various clinical appearances:

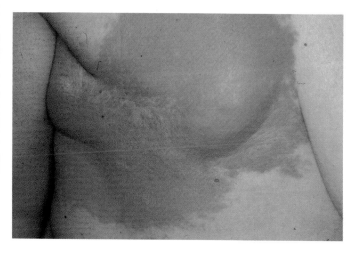

Carcinomatous lymphangitis
Classically observed in cancer of the breast, characterized by an extensive inflammatory plaque, sometimes wrongly called "carcinomatous erysipelas".

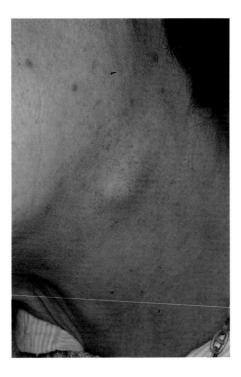

Nodular cutaneous-subcutaneous metastases

forming skin-embedded spherical colourless or bluish masses.

MELANOMA (MALIGNANT)

Melanoma is a tumour which develops either as a primary lesion from epidermal melanocytes or from the cells of congenital junctional and compound naevi, or much more rarely from intradermal and blue naevi. It metastasizes via lymph and/or blood. Several variants of melanoma have been described:

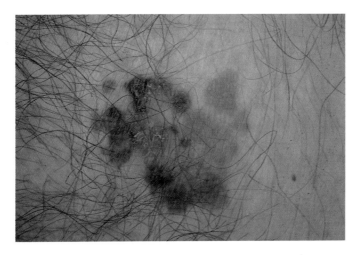

SUPERFICIAL SPREADING MELANOMA (SSM)

Slightly raised melanotic spot, varying in colour from brown to black, with a polycyclic margin. It undergoes a horizontal growth phase lasting several months and then finally starts its vertical phase, in which it invades the deep tissue.
It occurs anywhere on the body, but more readily on the back in men and on the legs in women.

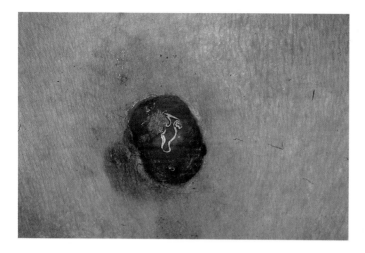

NODULAR MELANOMA
Infiltrated brown or black nodules, sometimes violet-red and more rarely achromic. The lesion, which is often dome-shaped, finally ulcerates and bleeds.

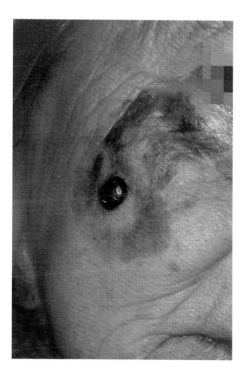

MELANOMA DEVELOPING OVER DUBREUILH'S MELANOSIS PRECANCEROSA
Infiltrated nodular formations, which may or may not be pigmented, sometimes oozing blood, developing from a Dubreuilh's melanosis.

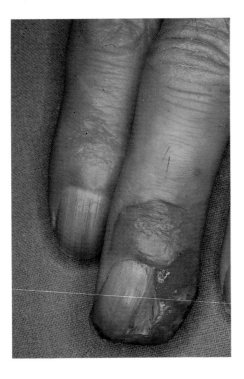

ACRAL LENTIGINOUS MELANOMA (MELANOMA OF THE EXTREMITIES)

Located on the extremities (palm of the hand, sole of foot, digital extremities), it resembles superficial spreading melanoma or nodular melanoma, representing only a particular site of either of these. The illustration suggests this double categorization particularly well.

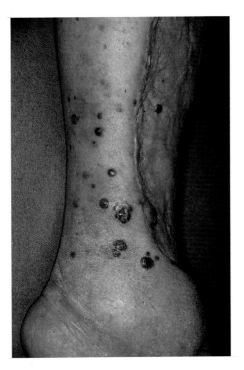

MELANOMA METASTASES

Numerous black or bluish indurated nodules developing near a previously excised melanoma.

DERMATOFIBROSARCOMA PROTUBERANS (DARIER-FERRAND FIBROSARCOMA)

Large multinodular dented tumour which adheres to the skin surface without ulcerating it and infiltrates the dermis and subcutaneous tissue, often beyond the limits of palpation. The tumour develops gradually, without painful symptoms. It affects adults of both sexes with a preference for the trunk and the base of the limbs. This fibrosarcoma has local malignancy, but can metastasize in exceptional cases.

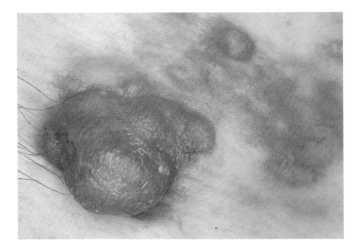

KAPOSI'S ANGIOSARCOMA

Violet nodules on the ankles and feet in an elderly patient. In the present case it is not occurring in the context of acquired immune deficiency syndrome.

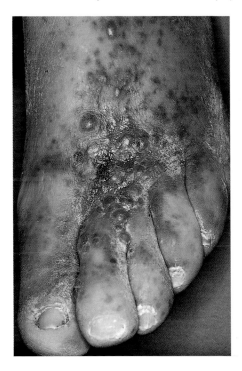

MALIGNANT LYMPHOMAS - MYCOSIS FUNGOIDES

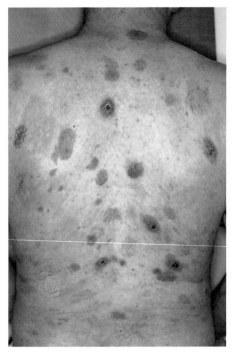

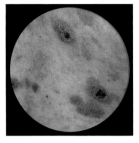

Among the many malignant cutaneous lymphomas, mycosis fungoides (epidermotropic T-lymphoma) represents an unusual entity. At the eruptive stage the clinical picture is characterized by dull coppery red infiltrated plaques distributed in arcs (photo 1). Tumours can subsequently develop, and these may ulcerate (photo 2).

photo 1

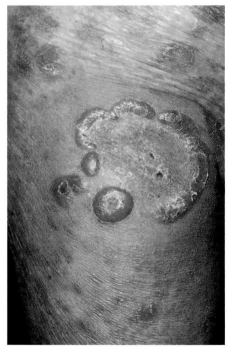

photo 2

PARANEOPLASTIC SYNDROMES

Malignant neoplasms can be accompanied by skin diseases which themselves are not neoplastic in character, nor directly caused by the presence of the tumour (in contrast to metastases), but which develop alongside the malignant neoplasm, regressing if and when the latter is eliminated and reappearing if it recurs. These so-called paraneoplastic dermatoses can occur when the malignant neoplasm has already distinctly developed, but they can also appear as a sign revealing a small neoplasm (Bazex's sign).

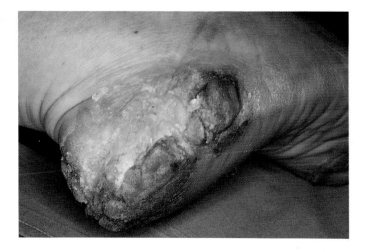

BAZEX'S PARANEOPLASTIC ACROKERATOSIS

Paraneoplastic skin diseases are, amongst others, malignant acanthosis nigricans, Gammel's erythema gyratum repens, and Bazex's paraneoplastic keratosis, hypertrichosis lanuginosa.
Both last diseases have been selected to illustrate paraneoplastic syndromes.

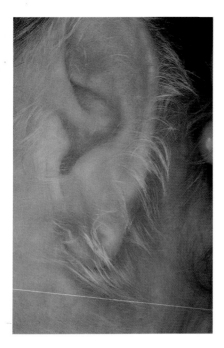

photo 1

HYPERTRICHOSIS LANUGINOSA

This occurs suddenly (within a few weeks), in the form of a down of long, white, silky, fine, and extremely numerous lanuginous hairs (photo 1) extending all over the glabrous skin and especially on the face. The rate of growth is accelerated and the hair (of the head) becomes more luxuriant. The papillae on the lingual mucosa are hypertrophic and glazed (photo 2). There is a distinct change in the sense of taste.

The appearance of such a picture must lead one to suspect the presence of an associated neoplasm. In the present case a neoplasm was detected in the breast. Radical treatment of the cancer leads to the disappearance of the acquired lanuginous hypertrophy. The recurrence of the neoplasm is accompanied by reappearance of the hypertrichosis (paraneoplastic dermatosis in the strict sense).

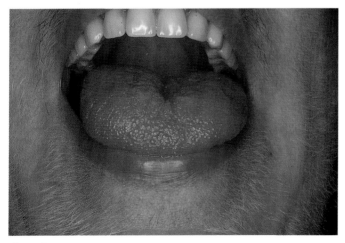

photo 2

ALGORITHMIC APPROACH
TO A
DERMATOLOGICAL DIAGNOSIS

**To conclude this pictorial prese
diseases for the general prac
interesting to include the m
dermatology applied to an every**

URTICARIA

PHYSICAL
URTICARIA?

NO

YES

PROVOKED BY DIRECT
CONTACT WITH A
SUBSTANCE?

NO

YES

OF GENETIC
ORIGIN?

YES

Simple or retarded
dermographism
→ rub with a blunt tip

Solar urticaria
→ photosensitivity test

Cholinergic urticaria
→ small papules induced
by heat, physical effort,
stress

Cold urticaria
→ test with ice cube
sheathed in plastic

Heat urticaria
→ test with test-tube of hot
water

Aquagenic urticaria
→ immersion test: hand in
water at ambient
temperature

Delayed pressure urticaria
→ test by pressure with a
weight strapped on to
the body

Vibratory angio-oedema
→ professional
circumstances
(particularly pneumatic
hammer)

Contact urticaria
→ rapid result patch test,
prick test or scratch test

Hereditary angioneurotic
oedema
→ investigate for
deficiency of C1
esterase inhibitor

URTICARIA REVEALING
HEPATITIS A

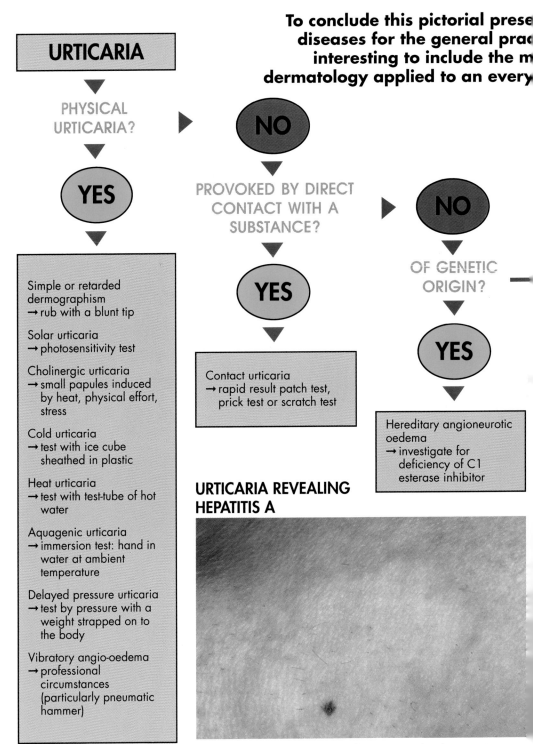

A quite exceptional case of figured urticaria revealing hepatitis A in its
initial phase. A raised semicircular swelling surrounds a central
oedematous, urticated zone, the very remarkable yellowish colour of
which is caused by accumulation of bilirubin in the oedema fluid.

ERMATOLOGICAL DIAGNOSIS

ition of the most common skin
oner, we thought it would be
ern diagnostic procedure in
y problem: urticaria.

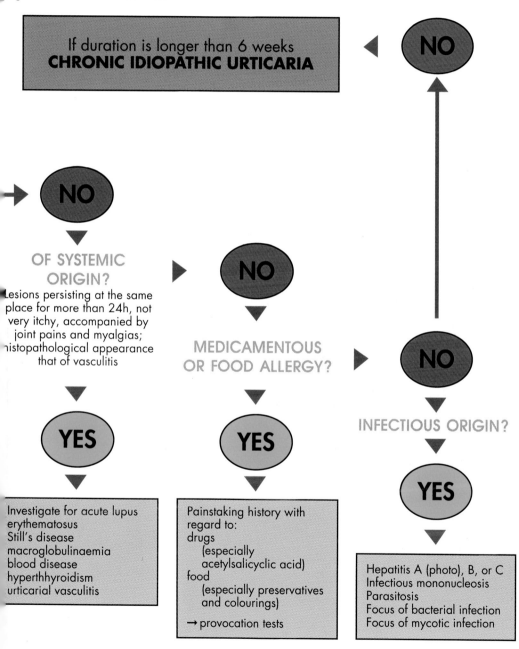

If duration is longer than 6 weeks
CHRONIC IDIOPATHIC URTICARIA

NO

NO

OF SYSTEMIC
ORIGIN?
Lesions persisting at the same
place for more than 24h, not
very itchy, accompanied by
joint pains and myalgias;
histopathological appearance
that of vasculitis

NO

MEDICAMENTOUS
OR FOOD ALLERGY?

NO

INFECTIOUS ORIGIN?

YES

YES

YES

Investigate for acute lupus
erythematosus
Still's disease
macroglobulinaemia
blood disease
hyperthhyroidism
urticarial vasculitis

Painstaking history with
regard to:
drugs
    (especially
    acetylsalicyclic acid)
food
    (especially preservatives
    and colourings)

→ provocation tests

Hepatitis A (photo), B, or C
Infectious mononucleosis
Parasitosis
Focus of bacterial infection
Focus of mycotic infection

Appendix to the algoritmic approach to the diagnosis of urticaria.

CLASSICAL DIAGNOSIS TO BE ESTABLISHED IN THE CASE OF CHRONIC URTICARIA IN ADULTS.

Clearly, a painstaking documentation of the patient's medical history combined with thorough clinical examination remains the cornerstone of the "diagnosis" of chronic urticaria in adults before the performance of any laboratory tests*. Laboratory testing, however extensive, will therefore be targeted, according to the answers to the questions received and to certain clinical peculiarities of the urticaria.

Even in chronic urticarias the classical medicamentous, food, and infectious causes must be sought with care. Before any laboratory tests all these possible factors, often acting only as cofactors, must be eliminated if possible, so that a further development of the condition is not encouraged.

For an adult patient suffering from chronic urticaria for which no particular orientation can be found in the medical history or the clinical examination, the following tests must be routinely requested as the minimum: blood count with total eosinophilia, erythrocyte sedimentation rate, fibrinogen, blood urea nitrogen, creatinine, liver enzymes, complete serology for hepatitis B and C, serology for infectious mononucleosis, cryoglobulins, antinuclear antibodies, Rose-Waaler test, latex test, complement C3, C4, inhibitor of C1-esterase, thyroid tests, total IgE, and possibly a few specific RAST tests.

Urinalysis and parasitological examination of the stool might be requested, depending on the results of the preliminary blood tests (e.g. kidney disorders or frankly pathological eosinophilia).

A skin biopsy with direct immunofluorescence may also be performed at this point, depending on the history and the clinical examination: suspicion of systemic urticaria associated with lupus erythematosus or of urticarial vasculitis.

Finally, it should be appreciated that the request for certain laboratory tests will often facilitate communication with the patient and thus help to gain his confidence. The doctor and patient can then cooperate in finding the most suitable treatment. Indeed, the psychogenic factors which may be responsible or partly responsible must not be neglected in the investigation of any chronic urticaria in an adult.

*Ann. Dermatol. Venereol., 1993, 120, 652
Reprinted by courtesy of Annales Françaises de Dermatologie.

INDEX